W0228032

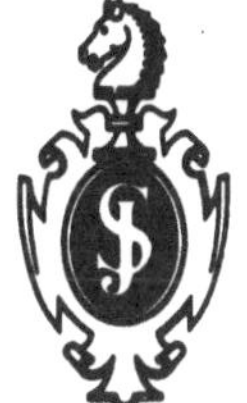

Philip F. Schofield, N.Y. Haboubi
and D.F. Martin

# Highlights in Coloproctology

Springer-Verlag
London Berlin Heidelberg
New York Paris Tokyo
Hong Kong Barcelona Budapest

Philip F. Schofield, MD, FRCS
Consultant Surgeon and Honorary Visiting Professor

N.Y. Haboubi, MB, ChB, DPath, MRCPath
Consultant Head of Department of Histopathology

D.F. Martin, MB, ChB, MRCP, FRCR
Consultant Radiologist

University Hospital of South Manchester, Nell Lane, West Didsbury, Manchester M20 8LR, UK.

ISBN 978-3-540-19779-9    ISBN 978-1-4471-3456-5 (eBook)
DOI 10.1007/978-1-4471-3456-5

British Library Cataloguing in Publication Data
Schofield, P. F.
Highlights in Coloproctology
I. Title
616.3
ISBN 978-3-540-19779-9

Library of Congress Cataloging-in-Publication Data
Schofield, P. F. (Philip F.), 1930–
Highlights in Coloproctology/Philip F. Schofield, N. Y. Haboubi, and D. F. Martin.
p. cm.
Includes bibliographical references and index.
ISBN-13: 978-3-540-19779-9
(Berlin: alk. paper): $28.00 (est.)
1. Proctology. 2. Intestines–Diseases. 3. Colon (Anatomy)–Diseases. 4. Anus–Diseases. I. Haboubi, N. Y. (Najib Y.), 1949– . II. Martin, D. F. (Derrick Frank), 1948– . III. Title. [DNLM: 1. Colonic Diseases. 2. Rectal Diseases. WI 520 S367h 1993]
RC864.S36 1993
616.3'4–dc20
DNLM/DLC
for Library of Congress    93–17623



Typeset by The Electronic Book Factory Ltd, Fife, Scotland

28/3830–543210 Printed on acid-free paper

# Preface

The medical world is getting ever more complex and the medical literature is expanding every year. These facts mean that the generalist in medicine, surgery, radiology or histopathology has begun to disappear. We have seen specialisation within internal medicine with the emergence of the medical gastroenterologist. General surgery has begun to fragment and surgeons with a particular interest in gastroenterology in general, hepato-biliary surgery or coloproctology have emerged and are now commonplace. The process is more advanced in the United States but a similar pattern is emerging in the United Kingdom and other countries. Similarly, radiologists and pathologists with particular or exclusive interest in gastroenterology exist worldwide. This catharsis has led in some institutions, including our own, to a realignment where there is a particular interest in gastroenterology because the basic disciplines have common interest and share the management of clinical problems. We have felt that it would be advantageous to bring expertise in gastroenterology from different disciplines together to write a book but to approach it from a different viewpoint to the orthodox text. Our aim is to take the key areas in coloproctology and select those references which are original and clearly written which led to the present state of knowledge and put these together with a summary of the present perceived wisdom as culled from these seminal references. We have included sections on the small intestine because many large bowel diseases also affect the small intestine.

We hope that this will be of value to the trainee who aims to have a good knowledge of coloproctology whether he or she aspires to be physician, surgeon, radiologist or pathologist. One aim of this work is to give ready access to the complex literature to those trainees preparing for higher examinations. We further hope that this method of presentation may help the established practitioner to see the subjects within coloproctology in a broad context drawing as it does from the experience of the allied disciplines. How successful we have been in achieving these objectives will be for the reader to judge.

Manchester, 1993

Philip F. Schofield
N.Y. Haboubi
D.F. Martin

# Acknowledgements

The authors would like to acknowledge the valuable help given by many people to produce this book, in particular, Dr. Wendy Schofield, who spent countless hours producing the first draft and subsequently helping to check the proofs. Finally we would wish to acknowledge our indebtedness to Mrs. Melanie Hinde, BA, ALA, the Chief Librarian at Christie Hospital, Manchester.

# Contents

# 1 The Small Intestine: Normal Structure and Function

The small intestine is adapted for digestion and absorption. The various enzymes responsible for the breakdown of complex substances may pass into the lumen from surrounding exocrine glands or be produced by the gut directly. The small bowel in post mortem studies is 600 cm in length but is significantly shorter in life (Hirsch et al., 1956)[1]. The surface area for absorption is enormously increased by the valvulae conniventes and the villous configuration of the mucosa, well illustrated by Morson (1988)[2] who describes the four types of mature cells covering the crypts and villi of the small bowel, namely enterocytes, goblet cells, enterochromaffin cells and Paneth cells. Under high magnification the enterocyte is seen to have a brush border (Zetterquist and Hendrix, 1960)[3]. The mucous membrane with its villi and crypts stands on the muscularis mucosa separating it from the muscularis propria. In the submucosal layer there is a plexus of small blood vessels, lymphatics, nerves and ganglia. The vascular arrangement is well illustrated by Carr and Schofield (1984)[4]. Morson (1988)[2] indicates that the goblet cells are most numerous in the crypts and decrease over the villi. The enterochromaffin and Paneth cells are found in the base of the crypts. The cells ascend from this base to the tip of the villus rapidly, with cellular turnover being less than one week (Williamson, 1978)[5]. Griffiths et al. (1988)[6] show that all the cells from a crypt villus unit are derived by division from a single stem cell at the base of the crypt. Unusual differentiation from the stem cell can occur under the influence of an abnormal stimulus, for example, Wright et al. (1990)[7] show that mucosal ulceration induces the development of a cell which secretes epidermal growth factor – a potent stimulus of cell proliferation.

The mucosa and submucosa are surrounded by smooth muscle responsible for the onward transmission of the luminal contents which is modulated by nervous and humoral influences.

The gut has its own immune system which is represented by various immune-competent cells in and around the small intestine. This system consists of intraepithelial lymphocytes, lamina propria lymphocytes, aggregates of lymphocytes in the bowel wall such as the Peyer's patches and the lymph nodes draining the bowel (Morson, 1988)[2].

Finally, the small bowel contains bacteria. The colonisation starts shortly after birth but the flora becomes established by the third or fourth week of life and remains relatively stable thereafter (Donaldson and Toskes, 1983)[8]. In health the stomach and duodenum are essentially sterile but in the jejunum there are low concentrations of gram-positive facultative organisms such as lactobacillus: the concentration rarely exceeds $10^4$ organisms per millilitre

(Gorbach, 1971)[9]. In the distal small bowel there is an increased concentration, perhaps up to $10^9$ organisms per millilitre and this flora contains coliforms and bacteroides species. The colon contains a much greater number of organisms, predominantly anaerobes (Sykes et al., 1976)[10].

The interrelationship between absorption, secretion, enzymes, motility, hormone production, neural influences, immunological factors and bacteriology provides a complex system for the maintenance of normal small bowel function. The situation is complicated because in disease the basic abnormality often leads to changes in the other functions (Russell, 1985)[11]. The literature about the normal intestine is massive and cannot be fully reviewed in a book predominantly devoted to clinical matters but some major papers should perhaps be highlighted.

## The Enterocyte

The enterocytes are important cells of digestion, absorption and secretion. Miller and Crane (1961)[12] localised the enzymes sucrase and maltase in the brush border. Triadou et al. (1983)[13] investigated the distribution of the disaccharidases and peptidases and found that although lactase and sucrase levels were highest in the jejunum, peptidase levels increased in the ileum. Fondacaro (1986)[14] gives a detailed description of intestinal absorption and secretion with particular reference to the mechanisms of control. Holmes and Lobley (1989)[15] review the expanded knowledge of the enterocyte and brush border. They identify 22 enzymes: disaccharidases and peptidases in the main plus 19 transport or binding functions localised to the brush border. Thus the primary functions of the brush border are related to digestion and absorption of nutrients. The mechanism of absorption is active and in many instances requires the co-transport of sodium ions. Most substances are absorbed by active transport in the upper small bowel but vitamin $B_{12}$ and bile salts have unusual mechanisms of absorption localised in the ileum. Schjonsby (1989)[16] reviews the present situation for vitamin $B_{12}$. In a few substances, absorption is purely passive by the process of permeation between the enterocytes (Menzies, 1984)[17].

## Enterochromaffin Cells and Hormone Production

The gut endocrine cells share with special cells in other organs a number of histochemical and ultrastructural characteristics. These cells are found in the thyroid, the pancreas, the pituitary, the hypothalamus, the carotid body, the adrenal medulla, sympathetic ganglia and the bronchus. The important histochemical property common to these cells is their capacity for uptake and decarboxylation of a number of aromatic amines and their precursors, hence the term APUD as an acronym (Pearse, 1974)[18]. It is widely accepted that these cells are derived embryologically from the neural crest (Weichert, 1970)[19] but Sidhu (1979)[20] suggests that they may develop from immature stem cells of the gastrointestinal tract which are capable of differentiating into mucous, endocrine, or other types of cell.

The gut is an enormous endocrine organ responsible for the production of many peptides and amines which have a trophic action on the mucosa and influence motility, secretion, absorption and blood flow (Bloom and Polak, 1981)[21]. Although the enteroendocrine cells represent less than 1% of the cells of the intestinal mucosa they produce at least 15 different families of hormones (Brenner, 1991)[22]. Endocrine cells are called enterochromaffin or Kultschitzky cells, referring to the person who publicised their presence; in fact they were first observed by Heidenhaim (1870)[23]. Although these cells look homogeneous and monotonous on light microscopy, histochemically they prove to be a constellation of functionally heterogeneous cell types, each with a specific secretory product. Each endocrine cell type synthesises, stores and secretes a specific polypeptide hormone and/or biogenic amine that acts as a chemical messenger in orchestrating the various functions of the gut (O'Brien and Dayal, 1981)[24]. The gut hormones have specific distribution: they may be mainly pancreatic – pancreatic polypeptide (PP), mainly upper intestinal – cholecystokinin (CCK) and secretin, or mainly ileal – enteroglucagon and polypeptide YY. They may be confined to the mucosal endocrine cells – neurotensin and motilin, or may be in the nerve cells and plexuses – vasoactive intestinal polypeptide (VIP), or they may be found in both these sites – somatostatin, 5-hydroxytryptamine (5-HT) (Ferri et al., 1987)[25]. Similar cells in the stomach produce gastrin, somatostatin, 5-HT, VIP, and enteroglucagon. In the large intestine there is enteroglucagon, somatostatin, 5-HT, VIP and PP (Larson, 1979)[26]. The regulatory peptides are synthesised from larger precursors by proteolytic processing and this is reviewed by Andrews et al. (1987)[27]. Dockray (1990)[28] reviews the regulatory peptides and points out that the stimulus to their release is by distension or nutrients in the gut or autonomic stimulation. The regulatory peptides exert their effects by binding to receptors on the cell surface. Although there is a vast literature, the exact physiological role of the endocrine and paracrine systems is still poorly understood. Dockray further discusses agonists and antagonists. Of all the gut hormones, somatostatin has attracted the most attention so it is of interest that Gorden et al. (1989)[29] have reviewed the action of somatostatin and its synthetic agonist SMS 201–995.

## Immune System

Marsh (1987)[30] reviews this subject in a book entitled "Immunopathology of the Small Intestine". Dobbins (1986)[31] gives a comprehensive review of the intraepithelial lymphocytes which are shown to be of the cytotoxic suppressor type. It has been demonstrated that both T and B cells from the gut will circulate and then repopulate the epithelium and lamina propria of the small bowel. Spencer et al. (1986)[32] examined Peyer's patches from the terminal ileum and mapped the T and B cell distribution within them. The B cells contain a higher proportion of IgA-producing cells when compared with splenic B cells (Woloschak, 1986)[33]. Mestecky (1987)[34] points out that the mucosa-associated lymphoid tissue (MALT) contains more lymphocytes and plasma cells than any other organ and that the primary function of MALT is to prevent dietary antigens or organisms invading the body. He points out that MALT is the defence system not only for the gut but also of the respiratory and genitourinary systems and that the most important immunoglobulin is IgA with IgM also involved. He also notes that local stimulus to MALT will produce circulating lymphocytes which will home back to the site of original stimulation and distant mucosae. Doe (1989)[35] presents a short review of the present position including information on the induction of lymphokine production as part of the T cell response.

## Goblet Cells

Goblet cells have been shown to produce mucus from the Golgi apparatus (Phillips et al., 1984)[36]. Allen et al. (1982)[37] point out that the mucin is characterised by its glycoproteins which are of enormous size and extensively glycosylated, leading to distinctive physicochemical properties. In addition to the protein and sugar chains the mucins contain varying amounts of sialic acid (neuraminic acid) and sulphate which contribute to the charge on the mucin and are important in resisting bacterial attack (Mian et al., 1979)[38]. Mucus produced in the small intestine is sialylated (sialomucin) but much of the colonic mucus is sulphated (sulphomucin). The chemical nature of the mucus varies in health and disease and may be important in relationship to the pathogenesis of some diseases.

## Paneth Cells

The function of the Paneth cells is unknown but Elmes et al. (1984)[39] found that the Paneth cell area was larger if the mucosal aspect of the bowel was sterile rather than if it was non-sterile. They felt that the cells had an antibacterial role.

# References

1. Hirsch J, Ahrens EH, Blankenhorn DH (1956) Measurement of the human intestinal length in vivo and some causes of variation. Gastroenterology 31:274–284
2. Morson BC (1988) Colour atlas of gastrointestinal pathology. Oxford University Press, Oxford, pp 94–97
3. Zetterquist H, Hendrix TR (1960) A preliminary note on an ultrastructural abnormality of the intestinal epithelium in adult celiac disease (non-tropical sprue) which is reversed by a gluten-free diet. Bull Johns Hopkins Hosp 106:240–249
4. Carr ND, Schofield PF (1984) The colonic microcirculation. In: Coloproctology. J-C. Givel & F. Saegesser (eds). Springer, Berlin, Heidelberg, New York, pp 11–25
5. Williamson RCN (1978) Intestinal adaptation. N Engl J Med 298:1393–1444
6. Griffiths FD, Davies SJ, Williams D, Williams GT, Williams ED (1988) Demonstration of somatic mutation and colonic crypt clonality by X-linked enzyme histochemistry. Nature 333:461–463
7. Wright NA, Pike C, Elia G (1990) Induction of a novel epidermal growth factor-secreting cell lineage by mucosal ulceration in human gastrointestinal stem cells. Nature 343:82–85
8. Donaldson RM Jr, Toskes PP (1983) The relation of enteric bacterial populations to gastrointestinal function and disease. In: Gastrointestinal disease: pathophysiology, diagnosis, management. M.H. Sleisenger and J.S. Fordtran (eds). Saunders, Philadelphia, pp 44–54

9. Gorbach SL (1971) Intestinal microflora. Gastroenterology 60:1110–1129
10. Sykes PA, Boulter KH, Schofield PF (1976) The microflora of the obstructed bowel. Br J Surg 63:721–725
11. Russell RI (1985) The small intestine. Curr Opin Gastroenterol 1:201–202
12. Miller R, Crane RK (1961) The digestive function of the epithelium of the small intestine. II. Localization of disaccharide hydrolysis in the isolated brush border portion of intestinal epithelial cells. Biochem Biophys Acta 52:293–298
13. Triadou N, Bataille J, Schmitz J (1983) Longitudinal study of the human intestinal brush border membrane proteins: distribution of the main disaccharidases and peptidases. Gastroenterology 85:1326–1332
14. Fondacaro FD (1986) Intestinal ion transit and diarrhoeal disease. Am J Physiol 250:G1–G8
15. Holmes R, Lobley RW (1989) Intestinal brush border revisited. Gut 30:1667–1678
16. Schjonsby H (1989) Vitamin $B_{12}$ absorption and malabsorption. Gut 30:1686–1691
17. Menzies IS (1984) Transmucosal passage of inert molecules in health and disease. In: Intestinal absorption and secretion. E. Skadhauge and K. Heintze (eds). MTP, Lancaster, pp 527–543.
18. Pearse AGE (1974) The APUD cell concept and its implications in pathology. Pathol Ann 9:27–41
19. Weichert RF (1970) The neural ectodermal origin of the peptide-secreting endocrine glands. Am J Med 49:232–241
20. Sidhu GS (1979) The endodermal origin of digestive and respiratory tracts APUD cells; histopathological evidence and review of the literature. Am J Pathol 96:5–20
21. Bloom SR, Polak JM (1981) Gut hormones. Churchill Livingstone, Edinburgh
22. Brenner DA (1991) Molecular and cell biology of the small intestine. Curr Opin Gastroenterol 7:202–206
23. Heidenhaim R (1870) Untersuchungen uber den Bauder Labdrusen. Arch Makr Anat 6:368–406
24. O'Brien DS, Dayal Y (1981) The pathology of gastrointestinal endocrine cells. In: Diagnostic immunohistochemistry DeLellis RA (ed). Masson, New York, pp 75–110
25. Ferri G-L, Adrian TE, Soimero L et al. (1987) Regulatory peptide distribution in separate layers of the human jejunum. Digestion 37:15–21
26. Larson LI (1979) Pathology of gastrointestinal endocrine cells. Scand J Gastroenterol 14(S 53):1–8
27. Andrews PC, Brayton K, Dixon JE (1987) Precursors to regulatory peptide – their proteolytic processing. Experientia 43:784–790
28. Dockray GJ (1990) Regulatory peptides of the intestine. Curr Opin Gastroenterol 6:246–250
29. Gorden P, Comi RJ, Maton PN, Go VLW (1989) Somatostatin and somatostatin analogue (SMS 201–995) in treatment of hormone-secreting tumors of the pituitary and gastrointestinal tract and non-neoplastic diseases of the gut. Ann Intern Med 110:35–50
30. Marsh MN (1987) Immunopathology of the small intestine. Wiley, Chichester
31. Dobbins WO (1986) Human intestinal intraepithelial lymphocytes. Gut 27:972–985
32. Spencer JO, Finn T, Isaacson PG (1986) Human Peyer's patches: an immunohistochemical study. Gut 27:405–410
33. Woloschak GE (1986) Comparison of immunoglobulin heavy chain isotope expression in Peyer's patch and splenic B cells. Mol Immunol 23:581–592
34. Mestecky J (1987) The common mucosal immune system and current strategies for induction of immune response in external secretions. J Clin Immunol 7:265–276
35. Doe WF (1989) The intestinal immune system. Gut 30:1679–1685
36. Phillips TE, Phillips TH, Neutra MR (1984) Regulation of intestinal goblet cell secretion. III. Isolated intestinal epithelium. Am J Physiol 247:G674–G681
37. Allen A, Bell A, Mantle M, Pearson JP (1982) The structure and physiology of gastrointestinal mucus. Adv Exp Med Biol 144:115–133
38. Mian N, Anderson CE, Kent PW (1979) Effect of the O-sulphate groups in lactose and *N*-acetylneuraminyl-lactose on their enzymic hydrolysis. Biochem J 81:387–399
39. Elmes ME, Stanton MR, Howells CH, Lowe GH (1984) Relation between mucosal flora and Paneth cell population of human jejunum and ileum. J Clin Pathol 37:1268–1271

# 2 Malabsorption

## Definition and Types

Malabsorption and maldigestion should be considered together and occur when one or more of the constituents of diet are inadequately digested or absorbed. Normal absorption is reviewed by Hegart and Silk (1983)[1] who discuss protein, iron and vitamin $B_{12}$. Caspary (1986)[2] and Heitlinger and Lebenthal (1988)[3] review carbohydrate absorption and Glickman (1983)[4] fat absorption.

A major review of maldigestion and malabsorption is given by Wright and Heyworth (1989)[5]. Malabsorption of fat gives rise to typical steatorrhoea occurring most strikingly in pancreatic disease. Malabsorption of carbohydrate gives rise to acidic, explosive watery diarrhoea and occurs typically in lactase deficiency. Malabsorption of protein leads to muscle wasting and oedema. Frequently small intestinal abnormalities lead to combinations of dietary constituents being inadequately absorbed and secondary deficiencies of fat-soluble vitamins (A, D, E and K) as well as vitamin $B_{12}$ and iron occur concomitantly. Deficiency disease may occur because of absent dietary factors, for example $B_{12}$ deficiency in vegans.

## Causes of Malabsorption

Conditions leading to malabsorption can be conveniently divided into intraluminal, intestinal (mural) and lymphatic (extraintestinal factors).

### Intraluminal

Malabsorption can occur when the small bowel is structurally and functionally normal but the luminal contents are abnormal. Examples include vitamin $B_{12}$ malabsorption in pernicious anaemia and steatorrhoea in pancreatic insufficiency or in biliary obstruction. Bacterial overgrowth for a variety of reasons may give rise to malabsorption.

### Mural or Intestinal Disease

There are a large number of diseases of the small intestine which lead to malabsorption. They include Crohn's disease, coeliac disease and Whipple's disease, various infections, radiation damage and rare specific diseases.

### Lymphatic (Extraluminal)

The extraluminal causes are all discussed individually elsewhere but include lymphoma, neuroendocrine tumours and tuberculosis.

## Clinical Effects of Malabsorption

### Fat and Fat-Soluble Vitamins and Calcium

Fat malabsorption itself is simply a reflection of underlying pancreatic, biliary or intestinal disease which leads specifically to deficiency of vitamin A, D, E and K and to calcium malabsorption. These are discussed by Romano and Dobbins (1989)[6] and their treatment and avoidance by Marotta and Floch (1989)[7]. Both these articles discuss the pathophysiology and management in nutritional terms of patients with malabsorption of all types, as does an extensive review article by Bickle (1983)[8].

### Vitamin $B_{12}$

Vitamin $B_{12}$ deficiency leads to megaloblastic anaemia, stomatitis, cheilosis, glossitis and in extreme situations to subacute combined degeneration of the cord. Malabsorption is due to intrinsic factor deficiency (pernicious anaemia or previous gastric surgery) or terminal ileal disease or resection. Vitamin $B_{12}$ absorption, deficiency, prophylaxis and management are discussed by Gallagher (1983)[9] who notes that in most malabsorption states this vitamin deficiency is predictable and avoidable.

### Folate Deficiency

Folate deficiency leads to megaloblastic anaemia and is usually due to jejunal mucosal disease. Normal and abnormal physiology are discussed by Gallagher (1983)[9].

## Protein Deficiency

Abnormal protein digestion and absorption are dealt with extensively by Freeman et al. (1983)[10] who discuss not only maldigestion and malabsorption but also inherited isolated amino acid transport disorders such as Hartnup disease and cystinuria. These authors list pancreatic exocrine disease and small intestinal mucosal disease as the main causes of protein malabsorption, which is clinically evident as weight loss, muscle loss and oedema. They discuss protein-losing enteropathy and its causes and pathophysiology.

## Trace Element Deficiency

Zinc deficiency can occur in malabsorption and is evident as dry scaly skin (acrodermatitis) and alopecia. Other deficiencies may occur, of copper or chromium for example, but usually only in severe chronic disease or in patients on total parenteral nutrition (Morris et al., 1983)[11].

# Tests of Malabsorption

Romano and Dobbins (1989)[6] suggest that the initial investigation of the patient with suspected malabsorption should include a full blood count with assessment of red cell indices, serum iron, ferritin, vitamin $B_{12}$, red cell folate, serum albumin, calcium, phosphate, carotene, alkaline phosphatase, cholesterol and prothrombin time. Normal results indicate that malabsorption is not a major clinical problem whilst abnormal results suggest malabsorption. They state that these tests allow malabsorption to be divided into two groups: those indicating fat malabsorption (low carotene, cholesterol, calcium and phosphorus), and those indicating malabsorption of water-soluble substances (vitamin $B_{12}$, folate, iron and albumin). Mucosal intestinal disease is a likely cause of malabsorption of water-soluble substances.

## Xylose Tolerance Test

The xylose tolerance test has been used to assess the possibility of proximal small bowel malabsorption although its use has diminished. Craig and Atkinson (1988)[12] indicate that the standard 25 g D-xylose test is more than 95% accurate in discriminating between normal and abnormal proximal small bowel. A 1-hour serum measurement, as opposed to the normal 5-hour urinary collection, was shown to be satisfactory in both the young and the elderly.

## Faecal Fat Measurement

This is a traditional first-line test in suspected malabsorption. Its use and limitations are discussed by Romano and Dobbins (1989)[6] who recommend 72-hour faecal collection whilst the patient is on a 100 g fat diet.

## Schilling Test and Variants

The Schilling test assesses the ability to absorb radiolabelled vitamin $B_{12}$ and theoretically is a useful method to distinguish between different causes of malabsorption. Abnormal vitamin $B_{12}$ absorption due to a gastric cause (atrophic gastritis) will be corrected by taking intrinsic factor. Pancreatic supplements will correct malabsorption due to pancreatic insufficiency. Antibiotic treatment will improve malabsorption due to bacterial overgrowth (diverticula, stricture, blind loop). None of these measures will correct malabsorption if it is due to terminal ileal disease or resection (Romano and Dobbins, 1989; Gallagher, 1983)[6,9]. Both these papers discuss the limitations and pitfalls of this theory and review the true clinical usefulness of Schilling testing.

## Small Bowel Biopsy

Small bowel biopsy is the definitive test in suspected proximal small bowel disease. Romano and Dobbins (1989)[6] review the range of possible diseases detectable on biopsy which range from parasitic infection (*Giardia lamblia*) to enzyme deficiency (alactasia), mucosal disease (coeliac disease, Crohn's disease) and submucosal disease (lymphoma, Whipple's disease). Scott and Losowsky (1976)[13] investigated the variation in appearance of small bowel biopsy in coeliac disease, finding some variation between duodenum and jejunum as well as between adjacent areas of jejunum. They recommend multiple biopsies from both duodenum and jejunum to diagnose the disease but more importantly to assess response to treatment. Duodenal biopsies obtained at endoscopy are an accurate method of diagnosis of coeliac disease and a normal biopsy excludes the diagnosis. Holdstock et al. (1979)[14] found that only 3% of 270 biopsies were technically unsatisfactory and conclude that endoscopic duodenal biopsy was an effective method of excluding coeliac disease in clinically suspicious circumstances. This was confirmed by Brocchi et al. (1988)[15] who also described the loss of circular folds in the duodenum characteristic of subtotal villous atrophy.

## Breath Tests

King and Toskes (1983)[16] reviewed the wide range of breath tests under evaluation at that time for the assessment of carbohydrate and fat malabsorption and for bacterial overgrowth. They concluded that the $H_2$ lactose was an effective, simple and safe method of assessing alactasia and that the

[$^{14}C$]xylose breath test was the most useful method of detecting bacterial overgrowth. They felt that the [$^{14}C$]triolein breath test to assess fat malabsorption was promising. Romano and Dobbins (1989)[6] note that longer experience with [$^{14}C$]triolein breath test has been disappointing and the clinical use of breath tests is now limited to $H_2$ lactose for disaccharidase deficiency and [$^{14}C$]xylose for bacterial overgrowth. Both these articles review the physiology and methodology of breath testing in addition to their clinical usefulness.

### Radiology

Small intestinal contrast examination is important when local pathology (Crohn's, fistula, stricture, tumour, neoplasm or previous surgery) has a part to play in malabsorption. The main problem of barium radiology is that slight small bowel dilatation, thickening of folds, breaking up of barium and reduced transit seen in malabsorption states are entirely non-specific in terms of underlying pathology (Clemett and Marshak, 1969)[17]. A splendidly illustrated editorial by Herlinger (1992)[18] stresses the diagnosis of unsuspected coeliac disease during radiological examination although it emphasises the view that radiology is non-specific except when structural abnormalities are sought.

## Coeliac Disease

Coeliac disease was recognised in 1888 by Samuel Gee,[19], a physician at St Bartholomew's Hospital, as a disease affecting children, associated with offensive diarrhoea and failure to thrive. Dicke et al. (1952)[20] noticed a reduction in the incidence and severity of coeliac disease associated with wartime deprivation of wheat-derived products in Holland, which led to the recognition of the causative role of gluten in the development of the disease. The development of peroral intestinal biopsy allowed the characteristic histological features of villous atrophy to be documented (Doniach and Shiner, 1957)[21]. It was soon realised that coeliac disease was not only a disease of children (Cooke, 1968)[22]. Holt (1985)[23] makes the point that it may first present in the elderly. It presents with an array of clinical conditions other than simply failure to thrive in the weaning infant (Holt, 1990)[24]. An interesting association is with dermatitis herpetiformis, a skin condition which has been shown to be gluten-dependent and associated with a gluten-sensitive enteropathy (Katz et al., 1972)[25]. Coeliac disease is associated with an increased risk of small bowel lymphoma and adenocarcinoma (Swinson et al., 1983)[26]. There have been striking advances in the clinical, biochemical, immunological and molecular understanding of coeliac disease in the few decades since its aetiology was described.

The genetic and molecular aspects of recent developments have been reviewed by Kagnoff (1990)[27]. However, the most impressive article on the molecular and immunobiological aspects of coeliac disease comes from Marsh (1992)[28]. In a 25-page article with over 250 references he discusses the history of coeliac disease, the chemistry of gluten and genetic factors. He relates the pathology including the immunopathology of gluten sensitivity and discusses the patterns of mucosal abnormality seen in the disease. In passing, he observes that the terms used to describe the degree of mucosal damage which are classically used are no longer acceptable and proposes a five-point scale of mucosal damage which, although not specific, is typical of coeliac disease. He also reviews the published evidence concerning the frequency of asymptomatic coeliac disease, particularly in relatives of patients and calls into question the current diagnostic criteria for the disease, which hinge on the demonstration of mucosal abnormality which reverts to normal on gluten withdrawal. Finally, he identifies areas still requiring elucidation and comments particularly on the need for further investigation into non-responsive coeliac disease, the underlying mechanisms of which are quite unknown.

## Whipple's Disease

This was described by G. H. Whipple (1907)[29] at Johns Hopkins University as a fatal disease of wasting with diarrhoea in adults with "deposits of fat and fatty acids in the intestinal and mesenteric lymphatic tissues." It is now recognised that the abnormal material is not a lipid. Although the disease principally affects the small bowel, lesions may be found in the lung, liver and in other organs. The diagnosis may be made by small bowel biopsy when PAS-positive macrophages are found in the lamina propria. Electron microscopy has shown large numbers of bacilli in the macrophages (Dobbins, 1985)[30]. This previously fatal disease responds well to a suitable prolonged course of antibiotics (Fleming et al., 1988)[31].

## Idiopathic Eosinophilic Gastroenteritis

Although eosinophilic infiltrates can occur in the oesophagus, stomach and colon, the small intestine is the commonest site of this disease of unknown aetiology (Blackshaw and Levison, 1986)[32].

Clinically the patients may have recurrent intestinal obstruction, perforation or bleeding (Morson and Dawson, 1990)[33].

## Intestinal Involvement in Generalised Disease

Collagen diseases and amyloid disease may involve the intestine causing disturbances in intestinal motility (see Chapter 16).

The gastrointestinal manifestations of the acquired immune deficiency syndrome (AIDS) are reviewed by Weller (1987)[34].

# References


1. Hegart JE, Silk DBA (1983) The small intestine. In: Recent advances in gastroenterology 5. D.A.Bouchier (ed). Churchill Livingstone, Edinburgh, pp 49–70
2. Caspary WF (1986) Diarrhoea associated with carbohydrate malabsorption. Clin Gastroenterol 15:631–655
3. Heitlinger LA, Lebenthal E (1988) Disorders of carbohydrate digestion and absorption. Pediatr Clin North Am 35:239–255
4. Glickman RM (1983) Fat absorption and malabsorption. Clin Gastroenterol 12:323–334
5. Wright TL, Heyworth MI (1989) Maldigestion and malabsorption. In: Gastrointestinal disease: pathophysiology, diagnosis, management. M.H. Sleisenger and J.S. Fordtran (eds). Saunders, Philadelphia, pp 263–282
6. Romano TJ, Dobbins JW (1989) Evaluation of the patient with suspected malabsorption. Gastroenterol Clin North Am 18:467–483
7. Marotta RB, Floch MH (1989) Dietary therapy of steatorrhoea. Gastroenterol Clin North Am 18:485–512
8. Bickle DD (1983) Calcium absorption and vitamin D metabolism. Gastroenterol Clin North Am 12:379–394
9. Gallagher ND (1983) Importance of vitamin $B_{12}$ and folate metabolism in malabsorption. Clin Gastroenterol 12:437–441
10. Freeman HJ, Sleisenger MH, Kim YS (1983) Human protein digestion and absorption: normal mechanisms and protein–energy malnutrition. Clin Gastroenterol 12:357–378
11. Morris JA, Selivanov V, Shelden GF (1983) Nutritional management of patients with malabsorption syndrome. Clin Gastroenterol 12:463–474
12. Craig RM, Atkinson AJ (1988) D-xylose testing: a review. Gastroenterology 95:223–231
13. Scott BB, Losowsky MG (1976) Patchiness and duodeno-jejunal variation of the mucosal abnormality in coeliac disease and dermatitis herpetiformis. Gut 17:984–992
14. Holdstock G, Eade OE, Isaacson P, Smith CL (1979) Endoscopic duodenal biopsies in coeliac disease and duodenitis. Scand J Gastroenterol 14:717–720
15. Brocchi E, Corazza G, Caletti G, Treggiari EA, Barbar L, Casbarrini G (1988) Endoscopic demonstration of loss of duodenal folds in the diagnosis of celiac disease. N Engl J Med 319:741–744
16. King CE, Toskes PP (1983) The use of breath tests in the study of malabsorption. Clin Gastroenterol 12:591–610
17. Clemett AR, Marshak RH (1969) Whipple's disease. Roentgen features and differential diagnosis. Radiol Clin North Am 7:105–111
18. Herlinger H (1992) Radiology in malabsorption. Clin Radiol 45:73–78
19. Gee S (1888) On the coeliac affliction. St Bartholomew's Hosp Rep 24:17
20. Dicke WK, Van de Weijers HA, Kamer JH (1952) Coeliac disease. II. The presence in wheat of a factor having a deleterious effect in cases of coeliac disease. Acta Paediatr 42:34–42
21. Doniach I, Shiner M (1957) Duodenal and jejunal biopsies. Gastroenterology 33:71–86
22. Cooke WT (1968) Adult celiac disease. In: Progress in gastroenterology. C.B. Jerzy-Glass (ed). pp 299–338
23. Holt PR (1985) The small intestine. Clin Gastroenterol 14:689–723
24. Holt PR (1990) Diarrhoea and malabsorption in the elderly. Gastroenterol Clin North Am 19:345–359
25. Katz SI, Falchuck ZM, Dahl MV et al. (1972) HL-A8: a genetic link between dermatitis herpetiformis and gluten sensitive enteropathy. J Clin Invest 51:2977–2980
26. Swinson CM, Slavin G, Coles EC, Booth CC (1983) Coeliac disease and malignancy. Lancet i:111–115
27. Kagnoff MF (1990) Understanding the molecular basis of coeliac disease. Gut 31:497–499
28. Marsh MN (1992) Gluten, major histocompatibility complex and the small intestine. Gastroenterology 102:330–354
29. Whipple GH (1907) A hitherto undescribed disease characterised anatomically by deposits of fat and fatty acids in the intestinal and mesenteric lymphatic tissues. Bull Johns Hopkins Hosp 18:382–391
30. Dobbins WO (1985) Whipple's disease – an historical perspective. Q J Med 56:523–531

31. Fleming JL, Weisner RH, Shorter RG (1988) Whipple's disease: clinical, biochemical and histopathologic features and assessment of treatment in 29 patients. Mayo Clin Proc 63:539–551
32. Blackshaw AJ, Levison DA (1986) Eosinophilic infiltrates of the gastrointestinal tract. J Clin Pathol 39:1–7
33. Morson BC, Dawson IMP (1990) Gastrointestinal pathology, 3rd edn. Blackwell Scientific, Oxford
34. Weller IV (1987) ABC of AIDS: gastrointestinal and hepatic manifestations. Br Med J 294:1474–1476

# 3 Congenital Abnormalities

## Congenital Lesions of the Small Intestine

Congenital small bowel obstruction presenting during the neonatal period is either intrinsic (atresia or stenosis) or extrinsic (malrotation or volvulus).

### Small Bowel Atresia and Stenosis

It is probable that duodenal atresia and jejunoileal atresia have different aetiologies because they show a different frequency of coexistent congenital abnormalities. For example, Down's syndrome is present in about 30% of patients with duodenal atresia but only 2% of patients with jejunoileal atresia (Nixon and Tawes, 1971)[1].

During embryological development, the duodenum passes through a stage when it is plugged by epithelial cells at 6 to 7 weeks. The duodenum recanalises at about 8 weeks of development and failure of this recanalisation may lead to atresia or stenosis. Traditionally it was held that jejunoileal atresia had the same pathogenesis, but Louw and Barnard (1955)[2] suggested that the pathological basis for jejunoileal atresia is focal ischaemia, usually due to volvulus. They supported this proposal by experimental work performed on puppies in utero reproducing atresia and stenosis. Louw (1966)[3] has produced further evidence to support his hypothesis and has shown that success after surgery for atresia is improved when the atretic segment is resected with an adequate margin. He feels that this is due to the removal of an area of bowel adjacent to the atresia which is poorly vascularised. Martin and Zerella (1976)[4] have proposed a useful classification for these conditions. Santulli and Blanc (1961)[5] described a variation on small bowel atresia in three cases where there was an anomalous mesentery. The superior mesenteric artery was obstructed near its origin and the dorsal branch of the artery was absent, leading to multiple atresias of virtually the whole of the jejunum and ileum. The ileocolic branch remained patent allowing the distal ileum and right colon to develop normally. Zerella and Martin (1976)[6] have stressed that this artery can be easily jeopardised during surgery to repair the condition.

## Malrotation and Small Bowel Volvulus

In an extensive review Dott (1923)[7] described abnormalities of mid-gut rotation, relating the anatomy to embryological development. He described the stages of normal rotation and the various anomalies that can result, emphasising with a description of three cases that volvulus of the mid-gut is the typical abnormality in the neonatal period. He emphasised an association between malrotation and exomphalos. He discussed the surgical management of volvulus and malrotation in the newborn, stressing the value of reduction with fixation to prevent recurrence. Ladd (1933)[8] discussed the causes of proximal small bowel obstruction due to congenital anomalies, including intrinsic duodenal stenosis and extrinsic compression from malrotation, often associated with abnormal peritoneal attachments between caecum and posterior abdominal wall or duodenum (Ladd's bands).

Louw (1960)[9] in an extensive review of the work of Dott and Ladd included his own experience to reinforce the views of these authors, but also felt that chronic and intermittent symptoms of proximal small bowel obstruction could be caused by malrotation and mesenteric bands. He described 34 of his own cases in older children and adults in whom intermittent proximal small bowel obstruction occurred. He described the radiological features of duodenal dilatation with associated malposition of the small bowel on barium studies and the effect of response to corrective surgery. Recently both Jackson et al. (1989)[10] and Gilbert et al. (1990)[11] in case reports, have reinforced Louw's belief that malrotation with chronic or intermittent obstruction can present with chronic symptoms including protein-losing enteropathy, pain and vomiting in older children or adults.

## Omphalocoele (Exomphalos)

Umbilical hernia is the most common anterior abdominal wall defect in the neonate but rarely causes complication and usually resolves spontaneously. However, omphalocoele, a large defect in the anterior abdominal wall covered only by amniotic membrane and peritoneum, occurs in 1 in 5000 to 1 in 10 000 live births. It is a defect of migration of the gut from the umbilical cord back into the abdomen and is associated with malrotation in the majority of patients and a short small intestine in some. The embryology of omphalocoele was described by Duhamel (1963)[12] who discussed 30 cases, 24 of which were simple omphalocoele containing gut and liver, 4 had associated diaphragmatic hernia and 2 had bladder extrophy. Nowadays, most omphalocoeles are detected by antenatal ultrasound although minor degrees may not be diagnosed until birth (Sipes et al., 1990)[13].

Hughes et al. (1989)[14], describing their tertiary centre practice of 46 pregnancies with foetal omphalocoele, found a 67% incidence of other congenital genetic anomalies, most commonly involving the cardiac, skeletal or gastrointestinal systems. Twenty-three pregnancies were terminated, 2 foetuses died in utero and 11 died at birth; 10 survived, most of whom were delivered by caesarean section. Survival was dependent upon the severity of the associated congenital malformations rather than on the severity of the omphalocoele. Sipes et al. (1990)[13] also found a high incidence (71%) of other congenital anomalies. Of 17 patients who came to delivery, premature labour occurred in 11 but 10 delivered vaginally without complication. This challenged the belief that foetuses with omphalocoele should be delivered by caesarean section.

In the child surviving pregnancy and delivery, the treatment of the omphalocoele is essential to prevent the complications of sepsis, torsion or rupture. Primary closure of the abdominal wall defect may cause unacceptable elevation of the intraabdominal pressure. Grob (1963)[15] described conservative treatment with local protection. This allowed epithelialisation in 40% but he found that 60% still required surgery. Gross (1948)[16] described a two-stage repair, closing the skin over the omphalocoele with secondary closure of the abdominal wall musculature after 6–12 months. Schuster (1967)[17] described a similar two-stage repair using Teflon sheets to repair the defect but also described a one-stage repair using Teflon in 11 patients, 9 of whom survived. However, the use of synthetic materials invariably increases the risk of infection. Yaster et al. (1989)[18] reviewed the indications for primary and secondary closure of the defect. The appropriate procedure is determined by assessment of the rise in intragastric pressure and central venous pressure (CVP) after a trial closure of the abdominal wall fascia. If the intragastric pressure is less than 20 mmHg and the CVP rises by less than 4 mmHg after primary closure then the procedure is safe. With higher pressures, a two-stage procedure is necessary. Yaster et al. treated 10 neonates successfully in this way, 8 of whom had primary closure.

## Intestinal Duplications and Cysts

Considerable uncertainty exists regarding the aetiology, embryogenesis and classification of duplications or cysts associated with the gastrointestinal tract. This uncertainty is compounded by the variety of terms given to these lesions: duplication cysts, enteric cysts, enterogenous cysts or neurenteric cysts. Characteristically the lesions are cystic, lined by gastrointestinal, usually gastric, epithelium and may have smooth muscle components in their wall. They may lie in either an intraluminal or extraluminal position. Lesions are most commonly found adjacent to the ileum but also occur in the mediastinum and, indeed, can occur anywhere in the gut from the base of the tongue to the rectum. They can occur distant from the tubular portion of the gastrointestinal tract, having been noted in the retroperitoneum by Dardik and Klibanoff (1965)[19] and in the pancreas (Martin et al., 1987)[20].

Bremer (1944)[21] felt that cysts arose embryologically in one of two ways, either by the persistence of a normal developmental diverticulum or by an abnormality in recanalisation of the gut. Persistence of a diverticulum would allow an intra- or extraluminal cyst to form on the antimesenteric aspect of the small bowel but, in practice, most cysts are found on the mesenteric border or within the mesentery. Faulty recanalisation seems unlikely because cysts are most frequent in the mid-gut (ileum) whilst recanalisation is now felt to be confined to the foregut and hindgut (see Jejunal Atresia, p 14).

A common point which has been made by many authors is that there is an association between intestinal duplications and spinal abnormalities.

Veeneklaas (1952)[22] proposed that intrathoracic cysts, because of their frequent association with spinal abnormalities, were in fact developmental defects due to the lack of separation of the notochord and foregut.

Bentley and Smith (1960)[23] felt that cysts in other anatomical situations were likely to be of similar origin and coined the term split notochord syndrome. Enteric cysts have been described within the central nervous system (Leech and Olafson, 1977; Malcolm et al., 1991) [24,25]. MacKenzie and Gilbert (1991)[26] proposed that the colloid cyst of the third ventricle is an example because of the histopathological similarity to spinal enteric cysts.

The clinical features of cysts are well described by Forshall (1961)[27]. Intrinsic cysts tend to cause intussusception or intermittent obstruction and present between 4 days and 13 years of age. Extraluminal lesions are more often discovered as an incidental palpable mass although obstruction may be the presenting feature.

## Meckel's Diverticulum

Three splendid review articles written three or more decades ago provide an excellent understanding of the lesion. Sloan et al. (1954)[28] quote the autopsy incidence of Meckel's diverticulum at the Johns Hopkins Hospital as 1% (103 in 10 000 autopsies) with 75% occurring in males. These diverticula had not been symptomatic. They found that the diverticulum occurred between 2 cm and 200 cm proximal to the ileocaecal valve (mean 80–85 cm) and was 0.5–13 cm (mean 3–4 cm) in length.

Embryologically the diverticulum is a remnant of the intestinal end of the omphalomesenteric (vitellointestinal) duct and is lined by intestinal mucosa in the majority of cases but by gastric mucosa in 20%–30% of cases. In 19 patients coming to surgery, the indication was haemorrhage in 6 due to an ulcer in the ileum adjacent to the gastric mucosal lined diverticulum, obstruction in 6 cases, intussusception occurred in 4 patients and perforation in 3. Sloan et al. commented that radiological demonstration of Meckel's diverticulum was unusual on barium examinations. This view was challenged by Berne (1959)[29] who reviewed the clinical features of Meckel's diverticulum and described the barium radiology with 4 correctly diagnosed patients before surgery. Weinstein et al. (1962)[30] analysed 162 cases operated on at the Mayo Clinic in the previous half-century. Most patients had obstruction, haemorrhage or perforation but he described 10 patients with neoplasms arising in the diverticulum: two were benign (leiomyoma), but 8 (2 carcinoid, 6 leiomyosarcoma) were malignant. They emphasised that Meckel's diverticulum can present in a variety of ways and needs to be kept in mind as a possible explanation of symptoms other than chronic anaemia in childhood. Artigas et al. (1986)[31] found that complications were more common in patients with ectopic gastric or pancreatic tissue within the diverticulum.

Jewett et al. (1970)[32] were the first to describe the use of $^{99m}$Tc-pertechnetate to image acid-secreting gastric mucosa in the diverticulum. Dixon and Nolan (1987)[33] showed that this investigation is not as sensitive as was initially hoped. In 49 patients with Meckel's diverticulum who were operated upon they found isotope scanning to be positive in only 1 of 5 patients in whom the diverticulum was bleeding. Angiography was positive in 2 of 3 actively bleeding patients.

Small bowel enema was performed in 8 and was positive in 7 and was felt to be the single most useful radiological investigation.

## Jejunal Diverticular Disease

Acquired diverticular disease of the small bowel is rare (Maglinte et al., (1986)[34]. Often the condition is asymptomatic but may give rise to bacterial overgrowth with malabsorption, which may be corrected by antibiotics. (Nobles, 1971)[35]. Surgical complications of inflammation or bleeding may occur (Geroulakos, 1987)[36].

## References to Congenital Lesions of the Small Intestine

1. Nixon HH, Tawes R (1971) Etiology and treatment of small intestinal atresia. Analysis of a series of 127 jejuno-ileal atresias and comparison with 62 duodenal atresias. Surgery 69:41–51
2. Louw JH, Barnard CN (1955) Congenital intestinal atresia: observations on its origin. Lancet ii:1065–1067
3. Louw JH (1966) Jejuno-ileal atresia and stenosis. J Paediatr Surg 1:8–23
4. Martin LW, Zerella JT (1976) Jejuno-ileal atresia: a proposed classification. J Paediatr Surg 11:399–403
5. Santulli TV, Blanc WA (1961) Congenital atresia of the intestines. Pathogenesis and treatment. Ann Surg 154:939–948
6. Zerella JT, Martin LW (1976) Jejunal atresia with absent mesentery and a helical ileum. Surgery 80:550–553
7. Dott NM (1923) Abnormalities of intestinal rotation. Br J Surg 11:251–286
8. Ladd WE (1933) Congenital obstruction of the small intestine. JAMA 101:1453–1458
9. Louw JH (1960) Intestinal malrotation and duodenal ileus. J R Coll Surg Edinb 5:101–126
10. Jackson A, Bissett R, Dickson AP (1989) Malrotation and mid-gut volvulus presenting as malabsorption. Clin Radiol 40:536–537
11. Gilbert HW, Armstrong CP, Thompson MH (1990) The presentation of malrotation of the intestine in adults. Ann R Coll Surg Engl 72:239–242
12. Duhamel D (1963) Embryology of exomphalos and allied malformations. Arch Dis Child 38:142–147
13. Sipes SL, Weiner CP, Sipes DR, Grant SS, Williamson RA (1990) Gastroschisis and omphalocele: does antenatal diagnosis or route of delivery make a difference in perinatal outcome? Obstet Gynecol 76:195–199
14. Hughes MD, Nyberg DA, Mack LA, Pretorius DH (1989) Fetal omphalocele: prenatal ultrasound detection of concurrent anomalies and other predictors of outcome. Radiology 173:371–376
15. Grob M (1963) Conservative treatment of exomphalos. Arch Dis Child 38:148–150
16. Gross RE (1948) A new method for surgical treatment of large omphaloceles. Surgery 24:277–292
17. Schuster SR (1967) A new method for the staged repair of large omphaloceles. Surg Gynecol Obstet 125:837–850
18. Yaster M, Scherer TLR, Stone MM et al. (1989) Prediction of successful primary closure of congenital abdominal wall defects using intraoperative measurements. J Paediatr Surg 24:1217–1220
19. Dardik H, Klibanoff E (1965) Retroperitoneal enterogenous cyst. Ann Surg 162:1084–1086
20. Martin DF, Haboubi NY, Tweedle DEF (1987) Enteric cyst of the pancreas. Gastrointest Radiol 11:35–36
21. Bremer JL (1944) Diverticula and duplications of the intestinal tract. Arch Pathol 38:132–140
22. Veeneklaas GMH (1952) Intrathoracic gastrogenic cysts. Am J Dis Child 83:500–507

23. Bentley JFR, Smith JR (1960) Developmental posterior enteric remnants and spinal malformations. The split notochord syndrome. Arch Dis Child 35:76–86
24. Leech RW, Olafson RA (1977) Epithelial cysts of the neuraxis. Arch Pathol Lab Med 101:196–202
25. Malcolm GP, Symon L, Kendall B, Pires M (1991) Intracranial neurenteric cysts. J Neurol Surg 75:115–120
26. MacKenzie IRA, Gilbert JJ (1991) Cysts on the neuraxis of endodermal origin. J Neurol Surg Psychiatr 54:572–575
27. Forshall I (1961) Duplication of the intestinal tract. Postgrad Med J 37:570–589
28. Sloan RD, Stafford ES, Singewald ML, Sinn CM (1954) Meckel's diverticulum. Am J Radiol 71:64–65
29. Berne AS (1959) Meckel's diverticulum. X-ray diagnosis. N Engl J Med 260:690–696
30. Weinstein EC, Cain JC, Remine WH (1962) Meckel's diverticulum: 55 years of clinical and surgical experience. JAMA 182:251–253
31. Artigas V, Calabuig R, Badia F et al. (1986) Meckel's diverticulum: value of ectopic tissue. Am J Surg 151:631–634
32. Jewett TC, Duszynski DO, Allen JE (1970) The visualisation of Meckel's diverticulum with $^{99m}$Tc pertechnetate. Surgery 68:567–570
33. Dixon PM, Nolan DJ (1987) The diagnosis of Meckel's diverticulum: a continuing challenge. Clin Radiol 38:615–619
34. Maglinte DDT, Chernish SM, DeWeese R, Kelvin FM, Brunelle RL (1986) Acquired jejunoileal diverticular disease: subject review. State of the art. Radiology 158:557–580
35. Nobles ER (1971) Jejunal diverticula. Arch Surg 192:172–174
36. Geroulakos G (1987) Surgical problems of jejunal diverticulosis. Ann R Coll Surg Engl 69:266–268

## Congenital Anorectal Deformities

Browne (1955)[37] made important contributions to the understanding and treatment of congenital anorectal abnormalities based on an understanding of the embryology. There may be a failure of migration of the anus or excessive fusion of the lateral folds producing a low abnormality, which is responsive to prompt but relatively simple treatment. The high abnormality ends above the levator ani and usually communicates with the posterior urethra in the male or the vagina in the female. This is an oversimplification and there is a significant number of variants. Santulli et al. (1970)[38] reported on a new agreed international classification in which 27 different varieties of deformity were recognised. This was simplified after a workshop held in Wisconsin in 1984 by using the terms high, intermediate and low abnormalities with a separate descriptive section for cloacal abnormalities in females. In addition, an attempt was made to standardise postoperative assessments (Stephens and Durham Smith, 1986)[39].

Although most of these variants are clinically apparent in the neonate, imaging may be helpful. For many years, lateral radiographs taken with the infant inverted were used to define the level of the abnormality (Stephens and Durham Smith, 1971)[40]. Ikawa et al. (1985)[41] have used computed tomography (CT) and this appears to give superior views of the pelvic viscera and musculature. More recently, Pringle et al. (1987)[42] have shown even better details from magnetic resonance imaging (MRI) and this is to be recommended if available. Boyd and Kiely (1986)[43] mapped the external sphincter and puborectalis by electromyography using a concentric needle and showed without question that there was significant external sphincter tissue in all patients with high anomalies.

Browne (1955)[37] described the treatment of the low abnormality by means of a posterior cut back and dilatation. He also described posterior transposition of the ectopic anus. These still remain the methods of treatment. For the high abnormalities, Kiesewetter (1967)[44] described a sacroabdominoperineal approach which involved dividing the fistula and bringing the blind-ending rectum through the puborectalis sling to an appropriate place in the perineum. More recently Pena (1985)[45] reported on his posterior sagittal anorectoplasty. After preliminary colostomy in the neonatal period he carries out the definitive operation some months later. In most instances he is able to accomplish the operation through a midline incision from the mid-sacrum down to the perineum. He employs a nerve stimulator to identify the external sphincter puborectalis complex. When the terminal rectum is exposed it is mobilised, tapered and pulled through the complex with careful layer-by-layer repair of the musculature. In only 10% of his patients he finds that it is necessary to add an abdominal phase to mobilise a high-lying rectum. The results of this procedure in Pena's hands appear excellent.

## References to Congenital Anorectal Deformities

37. Browne D (1955) Congenital deformities of the anus and rectum. Arch Dis Child 30:42–45
38. Santulli TV, Kiesewetter WB, Bill AH (1970) Anorectal abnormalities: a suggested international classification. J Pediatr Surg 5:281–287
39. Stephens FD, Durham Smith E (1986) Classification, identification and assessment of surgical treatment of anorectal anomalies. Pediatr Surg Int 1:200–205
40. Stephens FD, Durham Smith E (1971) Anorectal malformation in children. Year Book, Chicago, p 133
41. Ikawa H, Yokoyama J, Sanbonmatsu T et al. (1985) The use of computerized tomography to evaluate anorectal abnormalities. J Pediatr Surg 20:640–644
42. Pringle KC, Sato Y, Soper RT (1987) Magnetic resonance imaging as an adjunct to planning an anorectal pullthrough. J Pediatr Surg 22:571–574
43. Boyd SG, Kiely EM (1986) Pre-operative neurophysiological studies of the external sphincter and pubo-rectalis muscle in children with anorectal malformations. Pediatr Surg Int 21:184–185
44. Kiesewetter WB (1967) Imperforate anus. II. The rationale and technic of the sacroabdomino-perineal operation. J Pediatr Surg 2:106–110
45. Pena A (1985) Surgical treatment of high imperforate anus. World J Surg 9:236–243

# 4 Intestinal and Colorectal Injury

## Blunt Abdominal Trauma

Cox (1984)[1] indicated that the commonest cause of blunt abdominal injury was road traffic accident and it was often part of multiple injuries which required careful assessment and resuscitation. He indicated that liver and/or spleen were the most likely to suffer intraabdominal injury. Intestinal injury came next in order of frequency.

Dauterive et al. (1985)[2] discussing abdominal trauma noted that approximately one quarter of patients had evidence of intestinal or mesenteric injury. Hunt et al. (1980)[3] found that only 6% of these patients had intestinal perforation and this was much commoner in the small bowel than the colon.

Hughes and Samill (1962)[4] drew attention to late complications of abdominal injury. Winton et al. (1985)[5] review delayed perforation and Howard et al. (1987)[6] discussed late stricture formation. Paterson-Brown et al. (1990)[7] in an animal model examined the extent of injury necessary to produce perforation or stricture. Mesenteric detachment of more than 5.5 cm was associated with late complications and may give guidance in the human with regard to resection.

Polk and Flint (1983)[8] in a general review of blunt abdominal trauma suggest that perforation of the small bowel may be sutured or resected with anastomosis. They believe that colonic injury can be sutured in ideal circumstances but exteriorisation colostomy should be standard treatment for most cases. Fischer et al. (1978)[9] review the experience with peritoneal lavage. This is now a standard preoperative test to investigate intraperitoneal bleeding and has a better than 95% accuracy rate. Operation is indicated if the lavage is positive.

## Penetrating Injury

Thal and Shires (1973)[10] showed that not all patients with abdominal stab wounds required laparotomy. If the patient shows signs of shock on admission then laparotomy is indicated. For other patients peritoneal lavage is used and if this is negative, wound debridement only is required. Galbraith et al. (1980)[11] report that with this regime the negative laparotomy rate has been reduced to 3%.

Demetriades et al. (1985)[12] from South Africa, note that more stab injuries to the colon are on the left, presumably due to right-handed assailants. The paper reviews treatment in civilian practice. This includes antibiotic cover but the type of surgery is controversial. They favour primary repair in most instances.

Baker et al. (1990)[13] favour exteriorisation of the colon after repair as proposed by Okies et al. (1972)[14] and report good results. Polk and Flint (1983)[8] believe that where the injuries are multiple and complex, colonic injury should be treated by colostomy.

## Gunshot Wounds

There is a long history of different types of management but Cooper and Ryan (1990)[15] draw attention to the differences between battlefield and civilian practice. Such differences include type of weapon, the conditions for surgery, the degree of contamination and the delay between wounding and operation, and they point out that the methods of civilian practice cannot be safely taken to the theatre of war. Muckart et al. (1990)[16] say that most would agree that abdominal gunshot injury is an indication for operation but they believe that a small percentage of patients can be managed conservatively and they have managed 20% of their gunshot wounds without operation and without complication.

Fraser and Drummond (1917)[17] report a mortality of over 60% for colonic injury treated by suture in the First World War. Ogilvie (1944)[18] was able to show a halving of this mortality due to a policy of exteriorisation or resection and exteriorisation for colonic injuries in the Second World War. In the Korean conflict, Weckesser and Putman (1962)[19] adopted a policy of more rapid transport of casualties with better resuscitation and the use of antibiotics thereby reducing the mortality to 15%. Thal and Yeary (1980)[20] showed similar results in the Vietnam War. Steele and Blaisdell (1977)[21] in the United States were able to report death rates as low as 3% in civilian practice for colonic injury using the principles of war surgery, although they did treat a small proportion of patients by primary closure of the colonic injury.

Stone and Fabian (1979)[22] laid down criteria of suitability for primary closure of the colonic injury and found that it was possible to treat half the patients by primary suture with satisfactory outcome.

Morgan (1945)[23] classified the much rarer gunshot injuries to the rectum into extraperitoneal and intraperitoneal. Morgan noted the importance of considering the diagnosis in any injury to the buttock. Laufmann (1946)[24] reported rectal injury complicating 6% of buttock wounds. The intraperitoneal injury was treated by suture and colostomy with a low mortality. Lung et al. (1970)[25] in the Vietnam conflict suggested perineal exploration with removal of the coccyx to expose the rectal injury for repair and drainage. If the anal sphincters are damaged then primary suture should be employed if possible. A divided colostomy is mandatory. They employ delayed secondary suture of the skin wound.

In civilian practice rectal injury may occur due to perineal impalement due to a fall onto a sharp object (Goligher, 1984)[26]. Maull et al. (1977)[27] describe closed injuries to the rectum that may occur as a result of a pelvic fracture. Andrews (1911)[28] described the rectum or sigmoid lesion as a result of directing a jet of compressed air at the victim's anus. Raina and Machienew (1980)[29] remind us that the injury still occurs.

Schofield (1980)[30] discusses the foreign bodies found in the rectum, which are many and various, ranging from vibrators to baked bean cans and from light bulbs to tap assemblies. It is also to be noted that foreign bodies may lodge in the anorectum when taken by mouth and present as sepsis. Some of the foreign bodies are related to psychosexual disorders and may cause injury which must be excluded or treated. Sohn et al. (1977)[31] describes the injury arising from "fist fornication" where the clenched fist is forced through the anal canal. This can cause injury to the anal musculature or to the rectum itself.

Jones and Bass (1991)[32] describe perineal injuries in children. They fall into two groups: accidental due to falling astride or impalement, and non-accidental, largely due to rape or sexual molestation. Twenty-nine of these patients involved serious injury to the anal canal and/or rectum and they advocate primary repair and colostomy under antibiotic control.

## Iatrogenic Injuries

Christie and Marrazzo (1991)[33] review the situation with regard to colonic perforation associated with colonoscopy. They believe that the incidence is about 0.15% predominantly after the removal of a polyp by diathermy snare. They point out that patients who do not have signs which are diffuse or increasing, can be treated conservatively with antibiotics even if there is some free gas in the peritoneal cavity. They also recognise what they call a serosal burn in which there is local tenderness in about 0.5% of cases. These patients seem to settle satisfactorily in hospital on conservative treatment. Andersen (1947)[34] collected a series of injuries by rigid rectal instrumentation. The usual site of injury is in the upper rectum.

Enemas have been reported as causes of rectal injury. Large and Mukheiber (1956)[35] reviewed the literature up to that date. It is interesting that these injuries still occur as they are reported in the paper by Jones and Bass (1991)[32].

Full-thickness rectal damage is a rare but grave complication of barium enema. Savia et al. (1982)[36] suggest that there is a mortality of 50% for intraperitoneal injury but extraperitoneal injury, although still grave, carries a lesser risk. The diagnosis is usually obvious and is an indication for surgery with toilet of the peritoneum at operation under antibiotic cover.

## References

1. Cox FE (1984) Blunt abdominal trauma. Ann Surg 199:467–474
2. Dauterive AH, Flancbaum L, Cox EF (1985) Blunt intestinal trauma. A modern day review. Ann Surg 201:198–203
3. Hunt KE, Garrison RN, Fry DE (1980) Perforating injuries of the gastrointestinal tract following blunt abdominal trauma. Am Surg 46:100–104
4. Hughes LE, Samill GB (1962) Long-delayed complications of closed abdominal trauma. Br Med J ii:776–777

5. Winton TL, Girotti MJ, Manley PN, Sterns EE (1985) Delayed intestinal perforation after non-penetrating abdominal trauma. Can J Surg 28:437–439
6. Howard PW, Barrie WW, O'Reilly K (1987) Post-traumatic bowel stenosis. J R Coll Surg Edinb 32:124–125
7. Paterson-Brown S, Francis N, Whawell S, Cooper GJ, Dudley HAF (1990) Prediction of the delayed complications of intestinal and mesenteric injuries following experimental blunt abdominal trauma. Br J Surg 77:648–651
8. Polk HC, Flint LM (1983) Intra-abdominal injuries in polytrauma. World J Surg 7:56–67
9. Fischer RP, Beverlin BC, Engrav L, Benjamin CI, Perry JF (1978) Diagnostic peritoneal lavage: 14 years and 2586 patients later. Am J Surg 136:701–704
10. Thal ER, Shires GT (1973) Peritoneal lavage in blunt abdominal trauma. Am J Surg 125:64–69
11. Galbraith TA, Oreskovich MR, Heimbach DM, Herman VM, Cassico CJ (1980) The role of peritoneal lavage in the management of stab wounds of the abdomen. Am J Surg 140:60–64
12. Demetriades D, Rabinowitz B, Sofianos C, Prümm E (1985) The management of colon injuries by primary repair or colostomy. Br J Surg 72:881–883
13. Baker LW, Thomson SR, Chadwick SJ (1990) Colon wound management and prograde colonic lavage in large bowel trauma. Br J Surg 77:872–876
14. Okies JE, Bricker DL, Jordan GL (1972) Exteriorized repair of colonic injuries. Am J Surg 124:807–810
15. Cooper GJ, Ryan JM (1990) Interaction of penetrating missiles with tissues: some common misapprehensions and implications for wound management. Br J Surg 77:606–610
16. Muckart DJ, Abdool-Carrim AT, King B (1990) Selective conservative management of abdominal gunshot wounds: a prospective study. Br J Surg 77:652–655
17. Fraser J, Drummond H (1917) A clinical and experimental study of 300 perforating wounds of the abdomen. Br Med J i:321–330
18. Ogilvie WH (1944) Abdominal wounds in the Western Desert. Surg Gynecol Obstet 78:225–238
19. Weckesser EC, Putman TC (1962) Perforating injuries of the rectum and sigmoid colon. J Trauma 2:474–487
20. Thal ER, Yeary EC (1980) Morbidity of colostomy closure following colonic trauma. J Trauma 20:287–291
21. Steele M, Blaisdell FW (1977) Treatment of colon injuries. J Trauma 17:557–562
22. Stone HH, Fabian TC (1979) Management of perforating colon trauma: randomization between primary closure and exteriorization Ann Surg 190:430–436
23. Morgan CN (1945) Wounds of the rectum. Surg Gynecol Obstet 81:56–62
24. Laufmann H (1946) Initial surgical treatment of penetrating wounds of the rectum. Surg Gynecol Obstet 82:219–228
25. Lung JA, Turk RP, Miller RE, Eiseman B (1970) Wounds of the rectum. Ann Surg 172:985–990
26. Goligher JC (1984) Surgery of the anus, rectum and colon, 5th edn. Baillière Tindall, London
27. Maull KI, Sachatello CR, Ernst CB (1977) Deep perineal laceration – an injury frequently associated with open pelvic fractures. J Trauma 17:685–696
28. Andrews EW (1911) Pneumatic rupture of the intestine, a new type of industrial accident. Surg Gynecol Obstet 12:63–72
29. Raina S, Machienew GW (1980) Multiple perforations of the colon after compressed air injury. Arch Surg 115:660–661
30. Schofield PF (1980) Foreign bodies in the rectum: a review. J R Soc Med 73:510–513
31. Sohn N, Weinstein MA, Gonchar J (1977) Social injuries of the rectum. Am J Surg 134:611–612
32. Jones LW, Bass DH (1991) Perineal injuries in children. Br J Surg 78:1105–1107
33. Christie JP, Marrazzo J (1991) "Mini-perforation" of the colon – not all postpolypectomy perforations require laparotomy. Dis Colon Rectum 34:132–135
34. Andersen AFR (1947) Perforations from proctoscopy. Gastroenterology 9:32–43
35. Large PG, Mukheiber WJ (1956) Injuries to the rectum and anal canal by enema syringes. Lancet ii:596–599
36. Savia G, Volkmar P, Raoux M et al. (1982) Les perforations recto-coliques au cours du lavement baryte. Lyon Chi. 78:73–77

# 5 Infective Diarrhoea

The acute onset of diarrhoea may have many causes. The abnormality may be minor or major and may be in the small or large bowel. Diarrhoeal illness is a worldwide problem but the causes differ due to the hygiene and the environment in the location and the nutritional and immunological state of the individual. Acute diarrhoeal states are a major source of mortality in the developing countries (Wanke et al., 1987)[1]. The realisation that an oral glucose-electrolyte solution can be absorbed, even in the presence of diarrhoea, has made dramatic improvement in mortality in those areas where it has been introduced (Candy, 1984)[2]. Diarrhoea in the tropics is much more likely to be due to parasites such as *Entamoeba histolytica* than in the Western world where the majority of the infections in the adult are due to bacteria (Harries, 1982)[3].

In the Western world, the common bacterial infections are due to non-typhoid *Salmonella* species, *Campylobacter* species, *Shigella* and different sub-types of *Escherischia coli* (Loosli et al., 1985)[4]. Rarer bacterial causes are *Yersinia*, *Clostridium difficile*, *Aeromonas* and *Plesiomonas* species. Cook (1980)[5] discusses the types and mechanisms of gastrointestinal upset carried by food. There are three mechanisms that may be responsible for the acute gastrointestinal upset: (a) the food contains a toxic substance, e.g. certain mushrooms or a preformed bacterial toxin (staphylococcus);(b) food containing live bacteria which produce an effect by enterotoxin, e.g. *Clostridium perfringens* and *Vibrio* sp.; and (c) the food contains bacteria which are enteroinvasive, e.g. *Salmonella* sp. If there is an outbreak of gastroenteritis not only have the individuals to be investigated but the source has to be traced as a public health measure (Gilbert and Roberts, 1987)[6]. Gorbach (1987)[7] gives a good overview of diagnosis and treatment in bacterial diarrhoea. Many of these organisms can produce colonic involvement with demonstrable blood and/or pus in the faeces and sigmoidoscopic abnormalities. Viral causes are commoner in children and the commonest of these is rotavirus (Bishop et al., 1973)[8] but Norwalk agent (Kapikian et al., 1972)[9], adenovirus (Uhnoo et al., 1984)[10] and other unidentified small round viruses appear to be important, though they seem predominantly to cause small bowel diarrhoea. Other organisms, such as cytomegalovirus, are rare pathogens but major causes of infection in immunocompromised individuals (Jacobson et al., 1988)[11].

## Traveller's Diarrhoea

When people from the Western world travel to other countries, particularly tropical countries, they have an increased risk of contracting an infection and developing so-called traveller's diarrhoea (TD) (Steffen and Boppart, 1987)[12]. Dickens et al. (1985)[13] showed that it was not only food which carried a risk when they demonstrated that common pathogens could survive freezing in ice used for beverages. It must be remembered that non-infective causes of diarrhoea and colonic disease can begin abroad so that chronic inflammatory bowel disease and even non-inflammatory colonic pathology may present as apparent traveller's diarrhoea (Harries et al., 1986)[14]. Nevertheless, the majority of patients suffering from TD have an infection, usually bacterial but on occasions viral or protozoal (Steffen and Boppart, 1987)[12]. Infection with multiple organisms is not uncommon (Taylor et al., 1985)[15]. There is controversy about the possibility of prophylaxis. In general, most authorities believe that this should not be encouraged (Editorial, Lancet 1988)[16]. Dupont et al. (1987)[17] suggested that bismuth subsalicylate offered protection, reducing the risk of TD by about 65%. Reves et al. (1988)[18] suggested that prophylactic antibiotics were more cost-effective than treating TD. The problem with taking antibiotics is that if infection does occur, the risk of antibiotic resistance is much higher.

## Transient Colitis

Acute colitis occurring in a fit adult is usually bacterial in origin and stool culture may reveal the pathogen. However, a proportion of patients who have a significantly abnormal rectum associated with a sudden onset of colitis do not have bacteriological evidence of infection. These patients may have an acute self-limiting illness, so-called transient colitis or may have chronic inflammatory bowel disease at an early stage in its evolution (Mandal et al., 1982)[19]. It is important to distinguish these last two apparently inflammatory conditions because the prognosis and treatment differ. Further, it should be kept in mind that some patients who have pathogens isolated from the stool may have coincident chronic inflammatory bowel disease (Schofield, 1982)[20]. The pathologist has an important role in attempting to define the probable course and outcome in an attack of acute colitis. Rectal biopsy in a true acute colitis will show no features of chronicity such as crypt distortion, fibrosis in the lamina propria or metaplasia (Shepherd, 1991)[21]. Nostrant et al., (1987)[22] suggest that if inflammatory cells are seen between the epithelial cells but not in the crypts, this is suggestive of infective colitis rather than chronic inflammatory bowel disease. There is no doubt that distinction is difficult and it is best to repeat the biopsy at 6 to 8 weeks when the transient colitis will have reverted to normal histology as will the majority of the infective colitides but not chronic inflammatory bowel disease (Morson and Dawson, 1990)[23].

## Opportunistic Infections

There is a different spectrum of infection in the immunosuppressed individual so that opportunistic infections become common. In homosexuals there is a greater tendency to rectal venereal disease and immunosuppression leads to diarrhoeal states, termed the "gay bowel syndrome" (Kazal et al, 1976)[24]. Wexner (1990)[25] gives an extensive and authoritative review of bowel problems due to sexual transmission. He highlights the high incidence of gonorrhoea, chlamydia and herpetic infections of the anorectum in homosexuals, as well as protozoal, bacterial and viral infections of the colon. He discusses the colorectal problems of AIDS with colitis produced by *Cryptosporidium*, cytomegalovirus and other organisms, the increased incidence of lymphoma and Kaposi's sarcoma and the prevalence of anal warts and sepsis. It must be remembered that it is not only patients with AIDS that are immunocompromised but also patients after organ transplantation, patients who have had chemotherapy and probably the grossly nutritionally deprived in the Third world (Webster, 1987)[26]. There have been increasing numbers of reports of serious colitis produced by cytomegalovirus with severe symptoms and even perforation (Tatum et al., 1990)[27]. René et al. (1989)[28] reviewed diarrhoea in HIV-infected patients and found that the most common pathogen was *Cryptosporidium*, followed by cytomegalovirus, *Giardia lamblia* and *Mycobacterium avium-intracellulare*.

## Acute Ileitis

Sudden attacks of abdominal pain with diarrhoea and tenderness, mimicking appendicitis, can be caused by acute ileitis. At operation, there is a red, oedematous ileum but a normal appendix. This condition rarely, if ever, progresses to chronic ileitis (Schofield, 1965)[29]. It was suspected at that time that this was an infective condition but proof has been lacking. Puylaert et al. (1989)[30] analysed a series of 61 patients with acute ileitis and confirmed bacterial infection due to *Yersinia enterocolitica* in 21 and *Campylobacter* in 15 patients. *Salmonella* species were responsible for 4 cases. They were able to make the diagnosis of acute ileitis and distinguish it from appendicitis by ultrasonography which allows non-operative managment.

## Specific Infections

### Small Intestinal Protozoa

Stürchler (1987)[31] reviews the parasitic diseases of the small intestine. The major protozoa are *Giardia lamblia* and the Coccidia, both of which groups are associated with diarrhoea. Jokipii et al. (1985)[32] report a series of patients returning from abroad with both infections.

### *Giardia lamblia*

Halliday et al. (1988)[33] show that this protozoon takes up bile salts which stimulate its growth and protect it from the damaging effects of gastrointestinal juices. It is suggested that this explains its predilection for the duodenum. Infections occur throughout the world but are more common in Third world countries (Gilman et al., 1985)[34]. The infection can be carried by contaminated water and often gives an acute diarrhoeal illness (Jephcott et al., 1986)[35]. It is one of the causes of traveller's diarrhoea but it can also produce a chronic disease (Chester et al., 1985)[36]. The diagnosis can often be made by duodenal biopsy or aspiration. Boreham et al. (1984)[37] review the antibacterial chemotherapy.

### *Coccidia*

*Cryptosporidium* species is the commonest pathogen in this group and is a major problem in patients with AIDS (Cook, 1987)[38]. Nevertheless, it does produce a diarrhoeal illness in many persons who are not immunosuppressed, especially children and travellers (Freidank and Kist,1987)[39]. In the immunocompetent, the disease is usually self-limiting with simple supportive treatment.

*Isospora belli* is a less common pathogen and is usually seen as a cause of diarrhoea in patients with AIDS. They may be helped by trimethoprim-sulphamethoxazole (Pape et al., 1989)[40].

## Cytomegalovirus (CMV) Infection

CMV has emerged as a most important, opportunistic viral infection in patients with AIDS. Dieterich (1987)[41] points out that all levels of the gastrointestinal tract may be involved from the oesophagus to the anus. Jacobson et al. (1988)[42] report that the illness is systemic with mucosal ulcerations, most commonly in the oesophagus, stomach or colon. The infection responds to ganciclovir therapy. Kaplan et al. (1989)[43] point out that CMV can be a problem in other immunosuppressed patients when they report that almost 10% of their patients with heart-lung transplants have infection. They advocate early endoscopy for diagnosis because response to ganciclovir is good. CMV infection can also compromise patients on cancer chemotherapy and Spiller et al. (1988)[44] suggest that it can occasionally be a pathogen in the immunocompetent.

CMV enterocolitis can lead to perforation (Burke et al., 1987)[45] or toxic dilatation of the colon (Orloff et al., 1989)[46].

## Cholera

The story of Dr John Snow and the halting of an epidemic of cholera in the Soho district of London by the removal of the handle of the Broad Street pump, is well known (Snow, 1855)[47]. Since this established water carriage of the organism, public health measures have been able to eliminate the disease in the Western world.

Cholera is still a serious problem in developing countries and is a major cause of morbidity and mortality (Miller et al., 1985)[48]. The symptoms are due to the toxin of *Vibrio cholerae*, which binds to receptors on the enterocyte (Holmgren et al., 1985)[49]. The toxin causes activation of adenylate cyclase which causes sodium ion secretion into the gut and hence diarrhoea. Cook (1980)[50] describes treatment with fluids and antibiotics. Oral rehydration requires a glucose and electrolyte solution in large quantities but when depletion is very severe, intravenous rehydration will be required. Levine et al. (1988)[51] report on vaccines which were previously based on killed organisms. They report a vaccine based on living organisms attenuated through a recombinant technique.

## Typhoid

Typhoid fever is endemic in most parts of the tropics (Wicks et al., 1971)[52]. Cook (1980)[53] reviews the bacteriology and pathology. A severe form of enteric fever is caused by *Salmonella typhi* and less severe illness by *Salmonella paratyphi A*, *B*, or *C*. The infection usually comes from contaminated food. The organism is enteroinvasive through the Peyer's patches in the terminal ileum and leads to a septicaemia. It is several days before the typical ulceration in the ileum occurs with associated diarrhoea. In the UK the disease is rare and largely confined to people returning from overseas travel.

Mandal (1988)[54] reviews enteric fever and points out that the use of antibiotics, especially chloramphenicol, has transformed typhoid from a long, life-threatening disease into a short-lasting febrile episode with a mortality of under 2% in the UK. Although there have been reports of resistance to chloramphenicol, Mandal states that this appears to be relatively rare but newer agents such as ciprofloxacin show promise. Gupta et al. (1985)[55] report a series from India with a very high number of complications including encephalitis, myocarditis and perforation and haemorrhage of the gastrointestinal tract. The early diagnosis of enteric fever depends on isolation of the organism from the blood during the septicaemic phase. Rose and Abraham (1987)[56] point out that in Third world countries this may not always be possible but they analyse simple laboratory and clinical events and show that these can provide an accurate diagnosis in enteric fever. Archampong (1985)[57] reviews the diagnosis and management of small intestinal perforation in typhoid. He believes that the optimal treatment is suture of the perforation in two layers. If this is done, together with correction of fluid and electrolyte disturbance before surgery there is a considerable lowering of mortality.

## *Salmonella* Enterocolitis

The non-typhoid *Salmonella* species are one of the commonest causes of bacterial diarrhoea but most often it is characterised by an enteritis (Christie, 1971)[58]. Mandal and Mani (1976)[59] demonstrated distal large bowel involvement in some cases. This was the first demonstration that organisms other than *Entamoeba histolytica* and *Shigella* had a colonic effect. Day et al. (1978)[60] described the histopathological changes. Unless there are systemic signs, the condition is best treated by rehydration without antibiotics because they prolong faecal excretion of the organism (Asherkoff and Bennett, 1969)[61]. If there is evidence of serious systemic effect with salmonellosis, antibiotics are indicated. Systemic salmonellosis may lead to metastatic infection. There is an excellent review of the extraintestinal complications of *Salmonella* by Cohen et al. (1987)[62]. Cherubin and Kowalski (1990)[63] report that norfloxacin is effective in eradicating *Salmonella* from the stools of carriers.

## *Campylobacter* Enterocolitis

*Campylobacter* species are the commonest cause of an infective diarrhoea. It was not until 1977 that it was recognised as a pathogen and it was thought to produce an enteritis (Skirrow, 1977)[64]. Lambert et al. (1979)[65] showed that the distal bowel was commonly affected and the infection was difficult to distinguish from inflammatory bowel disease on biopsy. The disease is usually mild and settles on simple rehydration therapy. In more severe illness, erythromycin is the antibiotic of choice (McNulty, 1987)[66]. Weir (1985)[67] reported that by that year, *Campylobacter* had become recognised as the commonest cause of bacterial diarrhoea in the UK.

## *Escherichia coli* Enterocolitis

Levine (1987)[68] reviews the species which cause disease. Enterotoxigenic type causes diarrhoea in children overseas and is associated with traveller's diarrhoea. The enteropathic type may cause acute or chronic diarrhoea. The enteroinvasive type is a major cause of enteritis and colitis in children in the Third world. They are less common pathogens in industrialised countries. Enterohaemorrhagic *Escherichia coli* became recognised as a pathogen causing haemorrhagic colitis and the haemolytic uraemic syndrome as a result of investigation of an outbreak in 1982 (Riley et al., 1983)[69]. The injury is produced by a shiga-like toxin. Pai et al. (1984)[70] showed it was a much commoner cause of bloody diarrhoea than previously thought. Carter et al. (1987)[71] review the epidemiology and clinical spectrum.

## *Clostridium difficile* Enterocolitis

Pseudomembranous enterocolitis (PMC) has been recognised as a pathological entity which was thought to be due to low flow states (Goulston and McGovern, 1965)[72]. A few cases predated the antibiotic era but it became apparent that many cases were antibiotic-associated. Bartlett et al. (1978)[73] isolated *Clostridium difficile* from the stools of patients with PMC and demonstrated that it was the toxigenic strain of this organism which was associated with the disease. Since that time it has been apparent that most but not all cases of PMC are associated with *Clostridium difficile* toxins but this organism can produce a range of effects, from asymptomatic carriage through mild to moderate diarrhoea as well as PMC (Gerding, 1989)[74]. Although the clindamycin–lincomycin group of antibiotics were initially the particular antibiotics associated with PMC it is now well established that almost any antibiotic may be associated and in the United States cephalosporins seem to be the commonest. It is paradoxical that both metronidazole and vancomycin, which are used for the treatment of the condition, have been incriminated as causes (Bingley and Harding, 1987)[75]. In addition, antineoplastic agents may also induce PMC (Roda, 1987)[76]. There is also evidence of cross-infection in hospitals and other institutions. Testore et al. (1988)[77] highlight this in a recent report. The organisms produce toxin A and toxin B. The latter is cytotoxic and is the basis of the diagnostic test in PMC where the toxin is assessed by its cytotoxicity to HeLa cells in tissue culture (Larsen et al., 1977)[78]. Despite attempts to produce other assays, none has as yet superseded tissue culture cytotoxicity.

The histology of PMC was described by Price and Davies (1977)[79], laying emphasis on the summit or volcano lesion in the mucosa in the second stage of the disease. Gerding (1989)[74] reviews the whole subject with particular reference to detection and treatment. It is important to recognise that medical treatment with vancomycin or metronidazole is usually successful but there is a 10% to 15% relapse rate within a few days of completion of treatment (Gebhard and Gerding, 1988)[80]. On very rare occasions there are signs of peritonitis when subtotal colectomy with ileostomy may be required (Bradley et al., 1988)[81].

## *Shigella* Infection

The *Shigella* group is the classical cause of bacillary dysentery. *Shigella* has four species and 39 subtypes (Thorne, 1990)[82]. All *Shigella* species have the ability, controlled by specific genes, to invade colonic cells (Hromockyj and Maurelli, 1989)[83]. Colonoscopy has shown that the disease rarely involves the whole of the colon but always has rectal and left-colonic involvement (Speelman et al., 1984)[84]. *Shigella* isolates now commonly show resistance to multiple antibiotics and show the inappropriateness of prophylactic antibiotics (Panigrahi et al., 1987)[85].

## Amoebic Dysentery

*Entamoeba histolytica* worldwide is undoubtedly the most significant cause of infective colitis but it is largely confined to tropical areas. This protozoan parasite is said to occur in 10% of the world's population but only produces symptoms in about 10% of these (Cevallos and Farthing,1991)[86]. Weinke et al. (1990)[87] identify two high-risk groups in the non-endemic areas: travellers from the tropics and homosexual men. It is interesting that the organism is commonly found in suffers from AIDS but it is rarely a cause of the diarrhoea (Allason-Jones et al., 1986)[88].

Amoebic colitis often settles on conservative treatment with metronidazole but some patients show signs of peritoneal irritation, so-called fulminant colitis, when medical treatment has carried 50% mortality (Vijrabukka et al., 1979)[89]. Mtshali and Luvuno (1982)[90] showed that resection of the inflamed and/or perforated colon reduced the mortality to 24%. The same group now recommend ileostomy, repair or wrapping of any perforation with prograde colonic lavage and claim a reduction to a 12% mortality (Luvono, 1990)[91].

## Tuberculous Enterocolitis

Archampong (1985)[57] from Ghana notes that intestinal tuberculosis is still common in Third world countries. It is hypertrophic in the ileocaecal or colonic area but ulcerative in the lower small bowel. He believes that most patients require surgery as well as antibiotics because of obstructive symptoms. Haddad et al. (1987)[92] review the literature on the epidemiology, diagnosis and treatment and stress the need to remember the possibility of tuberculous enteritis. Anand et al. (1988)[93] advise intensive drug treatment and reserving surgery for the failures of drug treatment. Although the condition is much commoner in developing countries it is still seen in the UK (Schofield, 1985)[94]. Cases have been reported recently from the United States (Kasulke et al., 1981)[95] and Canada (Jacubowski et al., 1987)[96], which confirms the worldwide distribution. In the UK the condition is much commoner in immigrants from the Indian subcontinent (Klimach and Ormerod, 1985)[97].

Schneebaum et al. (1987)[98] described a chronic terminal ileitis due to *Mycobacterium avium-intracellulare* (MAI) in a patient with AIDS. It is now recognised that MAI is the cause of diarrhoea in about 6% of AIDS patients in the United States due to an enterocolitis (Gerberding, 1989)[99]. Hoy et al. (1990)[100] report good clinical and bacteriological response from using four antituberculous drugs in combination because of the known resistance of the organism to treatment.

## Intestinal Schistosomiasis

Warren (1983)[101] estimates that over 200 million people worldwide have some form of schistosomal infection. Three species of *Schistosoma* produce intestinal disease: *S. mansoni, S. intercalatum* and *S. japonicum*. *S. mansoni* is widespread throughout Africa, the Middle East, South and Central America and the Caribbean. *S. intercalatum* appears in Central and West Africa whilst *S. japonicum* is found in South-East Asia. De Cock (1986)[102], in an article in which he predominantly reviews the hepatic complications, gives a full review of the epidemiology, diagnostic methods and specific chemotherapy. The life cycle of the parasite through the snail, as the intermediate host, is described by Warren (1983)[101]. Chapman et al. (1988)[103] discuss the acute phase (Katayama fever) occurring a few weeks after infection. The chronic phase occurs months or even years after the infection and it is at this stage that the colon is involved. The eggs deposited in the submucosa can be seen but in about 20% of cases this progresses to ulceration and/or polyp formation with bloody diarrhoea

(Farid et al. 1976)[104]. Cook (1989)[105] reviews a series of papers from Third world countries which discuss diagnostic techniques and methods of control.

### Spirochaetosis

These organisms which are also termed *Brachyspira aalborgi* can be seen in the intestine of pigs. In humans, they are seen as a distinct, haematoxyphilic blurred, hazy, almost continuous line of microorganisms staining the luminal aspect of the epithelial cells. This abnormality is found in about 5% of patients attending gastroenterology clinics. It is seen in over one third of colonic biopsies in homosexuals (McMillan and Lee, 1981)[106]. The pathogenicity of this organism has been disputed and there are only very occasional reports which incriminate them as pathogens. However, antibiotics in some patients with diarrhoea cleared the organisms and resolved the clinical problem (Rodgers et al., 1986)[107].

## Intestinal Helminth Infection

Helminths are especially prevalent in tropical Third world countries but may affect persons from any country. Hookworm and roundworm (*Ascaris lumbricoides*) are the chief helminths worldwide (Stürchler, 1987)[108]. Anderson (1986)[109] has studied the factors which determine infection with helminths and the intensity of infection. Louw (1966)[110] noted that a majority of children in developing tropical countries are affected by *Ascaris lumbricoides*. Turner (1986)[111] reviews the dramatic improvement in treatment due to the development of the nitroimidazoles, benzimidazoles and praziquantel. In poor countries where helminths are endemic, the policy is to control rather than eliminate infection in the knowledge that better hygiene and living conditions are necessary for complete control (Stephenson et al., 1989)[112].

### Nematodes

#### *Ascaris lumbricoides*

Wiersma and Hadley (1988)[113] state that *Ascaris lumbricoides* are usually asymptomatic but may produce surgical complications especially in children due to obstruction. Small bowel obstruction may be treated conservatively in children or adults (Mokoena and Luvuno, 1988)[114]. On occasions, surgery may be necessary for obstruction, particularly if volvulus occurs (Wiersma and Hadley, 1988)[113]. Efem (1987)[115] indicates that perforation is not due to *Ascaris* and when it is associated it is because of some pre-existing coincident pathology causing ulceration and necrosis. Leung and Chung (1988)[116] discuss obstruction of the common bile duct causing jaundice or of the pancreatic duct causing pancreatitis and state that under these circumstances the obstruction can be overcome by removing the worm endoscopically.

### Hookworm

Cook (1986)[117] reviewed the clinical manifestations of gastrointestinal helminth infections. *Ancylostoma duodenale* is the Old world species of hookworm whilst *Necator americanus* is prevalent in most tropical countries not just the Americas. Patients with hookworm infection present with anaemia but the severity of the symptoms depends on the magnitude of the infection.

### Strongyloides stercoralis

The parasitology and symptoms are similar to hookworm. There has been continued interest in this because self-reinfection or persistent infection is common. The infection may have persisted from the 1939–1945 war in ex-prisoners of the Japanese, or in Vietnam veterans (Cook, 1987)[118].

### Whipworm (Trichuris trichiuria)

Bundy (1986)[119] discusses this parasite which occupies the ileocaecal region. It is responsible for a low-grade colitis which can lead to a failure to thrive in children. Trichuris infections are commonly associated with roundworm and hookworm infections (Forrester et al., 1988)[120].

### Enterobius vermicularis (threadworm, pinworm)

See p.146 for discussion

## Cestodes

### Tapeworms

*Taenia solium* (pork tapeworm), *T. saginata* (beef tapeworm) and *Diphyllobothrium latum* parasitise the upper small bowel. *D. latum* may lead to vitamin $B_{12}$ deficiency (Nyberg, 1952)[121]. The principal complication in *T. solium* is cysticercosis, i.e. dissemination of the ova via the blood stream with the formation of "cysts" in neural tissue. Treatment is by praziquantel (Richards and Schantz, 1985)[122]. Waki et al. (1986)[123] found that gastrographin, used to investigate gastrointestinal symptoms, causes passage of tapeworms, including the scolex, in many individuals.

### Hydatid Disease

Gemmel (1988)[124] reviews transmission of *Echinococcus* from the dog to its intermediate hosts, including man. Whilst this is a worldwide problem it is rare in the UK but the incidence in Wales is 20 times greater than the incidence in England. Other sheep-rearing communities such as country areas in Australia have a high incidence. Diagnosis of hydatid disease is based on immunological assays and imaging techniques. Marti-Bonmati and Menor Serrano (1990)[125] investigated the various imaging techniques in this disease.

Treatment of the hepatic lesion has been by surgery until recently but with more effective drugs the emphasis is changing to a combination of drug treatment with surgery or even drug treatment followed by aspiration and instillation of 95% alcohol into the cyst under radiological control (Filice et al., 1990)[126].

## References


1. Wanke CA, Lima AAM, Guerrant RL (1987) Infectious diarrhoea in tropical and subtropical regions. Baillière Clin Gastroenterol 1:335–360
2. Candy DCA (1984) Diarrhoea, dehydration and drugs. Br Med J 289:1245–1246
3. Harries J (1982) Amoebiasis: a review. J R Soc Med 75:190–197
4. Loosli J, Gyr K, Stalder H et al. (1985) Etiology of acute infectious diarrhoea in a highly industrialized area of Switzerland. Gastroenterology 88:75–79
5. Cook G C (1980) Acute bacterial and viral infections of the small intestine. In: Tropical gastroenterology. Oxford University Press, Oxford, pp. 225–243
6. Gilbert RJ, Roberts D (1987) Food hygiene aspects and laboratory methods. *Salmonella* special. Revision of PHLS Microbiology Digest 3:9–11.
7. Gorbach SL (1987) Bacterial diarrhoea and its treatment. Lancet ii:1378–1381
8. Bishop RF, Davidson GP, Holmes IH, Ruck BJ (1973) Virus particles in epithelial cells of duodenal mucosa from children with acute non-bacterial gastroenteritis. Lancet ii:1281–1283
9. Kapikian AZ, Wyatt RG, Dolin R et al. (1972) Visualization by immune electron microscopy of a 27-nm particle associated with acute infectious non-bacterial gastroenteritis. J Virol 10:1075–1081.
10. Uhnoo I, Wadell G, Svensson L, Johnasson ME (1984) Importance of enteric adenoviruses 40 and 41 in acute gastroenteritis in infants and young children. J Clin Microbiol 20:365–372
11. Jacobson MA, O'Donnell JJ, Porteus D et al. (1988) Retinal and gastrointestinal disease due to cytomegalovirus in patients with the acquired immunodeficiency syndrome. Prevalence, natural history and response to ganciclovir therapy. Q J Med 67:473–486
12. Steffen R, Boppart I (1987) Traveller's diarrhoea. Baillière Clin Gastroenterol 1:361–376
13. Dickens DL, Dupont HL, Johnson PC (1985) Survival of bacterial enteropathogens in the ice of popular drinks. JAMA 253:3141–3143
14. Harries AD, Myers B, Cook GC (1986) Inflammatory disease: a common cause of bloody diarrhoea in visitors to the tropics. Br Med J 291:1686–1687
15. Taylor DN, Echeverria P, Blaser MJ et al. (1985) Polymicrobial aetiology of traveller's diarrhoea. Lancet i:381–383
16. Editorial (1988) Preventing traveller's diarrhoea. Lancet ii:144
17. Dupont HL, Ericsson CD, Johnson PC et al. (1987) Prevention of traveller's diarrhoea by tablet formulation of bismuth subsalicylate. JAMA 257:1347–1350
18. Reves RR, Johnson PC, Ericsson CD, Dupont HL (1988) A cost-effectiveness comparison of the use of antimicrobial agents for the treatment or prophylaxis of traveller's diarrhoea. Arch Intern Med 148:2421–2427
19. Mandal BK, Schofield PF, Morson BC (1982) A clinico-pathological study of acute colitis. The dilemma of the transient colitis syndrome. Scand J Gastroenterol 17:865–869
20. Schofield PF (1982) Toxic dilatation and perforation in inflammatory bowel disease. Ann R Coll Surg Engl 64:318–320
21. Shepherd NA (1991) Pathological mimics of chronic inflammatory bowel disease. J Clin Pathol 44:726–733
22. Nostrant TT, Kumar NB, Appleman HD (1987) Histopathology differentiates self-limited colitis from ulcerative colitis. Gastroenterology 92:318–328

23. Morson BC, Dawson IMP (1990) Gastrointestinal pathology, 3rd edn Blackwell Scientific, Oxford, p 481
24. Kazal HL, Sohn N, Carrasco JI (1976) The gay bowel syndrome: clinicopathologic correlation in 260 cases. Am Clin Lab Sci 6:184–192
25. Wexner SD (1990) Sexually transmitted diseases of the colon, rectum and anus. Dis Colon Rectum 33:1048–1062
26. Webster ADB (1987) Immunodeficiency and the gut. Baillière Clin Gastroenterol 1:547–566
27. Tatum E, Sun P, Cohn D (1990) Cytomegalovirus vasculitis and colon perforation in a patient with the acquired immunodeficiency syndrome. Pathology 21:235–238
28. René E, Marche C, Regnier B et al. (1989) Intestinal infections in patients with acquired immunodeficiency syndrome. A prospective study of 132 patients. Dig Dis Sci 34:773–780
29. Schofield PF (1965) The natural history and treatment of Crohn's disease. Ann R Coll Surg Engl 36:258–279
30. Puylaert JBCM, Vermeijden RJ, Van der Werf SDJ et al. (1989) Incidence and sonographic diagnosis of bacterial ileocaecitis masquerading as appendicitis. Lancet ii:84–85
31. Stürchler D (1987) Parasitic disease of the small intestinal tract. Baillière Clin Gastroenterol 1:397–424
32. Jokipii AMM, Hemilä M, Jokipii L (1985) Prospective study of acquisition of *Cryptosporidium*, *Giardia lamblia* and gastrointestinal illness. Lancet ii:487–489
33. Halliday CEW, Clark C, Farthing MJG (1988) *Giardia*–bile salt interactions in vitro and in vivo. Trans R Soc Trop Med Hyg 82:428–432
34. Gilman RH, Brown KH, Visvesvara GS et al. (1985) Epidemiology and serology of *Giardia lamblia* in a developing country: Bangladesh. Trans R Soc Trop Med Hyg 79:469–473
35. Jephcott AE, Begg NT, Baker IA (1986) Outbreak of giardiasis associated with mains water in the United Kingdom. Lancet i:730–731
36. Chester AC, MacMurray FC, Restifo MD, Mann O (1985) Giardiasis as a chronic disease. Dig Dis Sci 30:215–218
37. Boreham PF, Phillips RE, Shepherd RW (1984) The sensitivity of *Giardia intestinalis* to drugs in vitro. J Antimicrob Chemother 14:449–461
38. Cook GC (1987) Intestinal parasitic infection. Curr Opin Gastroenterol 3:130–141
39. Freidank H, Kist M (1987) Cryptosporidia in immunocompetent patients with gastroenteritis. Eur J Clin Microbiol 6:56–58
40. Pape JW, Verdier RI, Johnson WD (1989) Treatment and prophylaxis of *Isospora belli* infection in patients with AIDS. N Engl J Med 320:1044–1047
41. Dieterich DT (1987) Cytomegalovirus: a new gastrointestinal pathogen in immunocompromised patients. Am J Gastroenterol 82:764–765
42. Jacobson MA, O'Donnell JJ, Porteus D, Brodie HR, Feigel D, Mills J (1988) Retinal and gastrointestinal disease due to cytomegalovirus in patients with the acquired immunodeficiency syndrome: prevalence, natural history and response to ganciclovir therapy. Q J Med 67:473–486
43. Kaplan CS, Petersen EA, Icenogle TB et al. (1989) Gastrointestinal cytomegalovirus infection in heart and heart-lung transplant recipients. Arch Intern Med 149:2095–2100
44. Spiller RC, Lovell D, Silk DBA (1988) Adult acquired cytomegalovirus infection with gastric and duodenal ulceration. Gut 29:1109–1111
45. Burke G, Nichols L, Balough K et al. (1987) Perforations of the terminal ileum with cytomegalovirus vasculitis and Kaposi's sarcoma in a patient with acquired immunodeficiency syndrome. Surgery 102:540–545
46. Orloff JJ, Saito R, Lasky S, Dave H (1989) Toxic megacolon in cytomegalovirus colitis. Am J Gastroenterol 84:794–797
47. Snow J (1855) On the mode of communication of cholera, 2nd edn. Churchill, London
48. Miller CJ, Feachem RG, Drasar BS (1985) Cholera epidemiology in developed and developing countries: new thought on transmission, seasonality and control. Lancet i:261–263
49. Holmgren J, Lindblad M, Fredman P, Svennerholm L, Myrvold H (1985) Comparison of receptors for cholera and *Escherichia coli* enterotoxins in human intestine. Gastroenterology 89:27–35
50. Cook GC (1980) Tropical gastroenterology. Oxford University Press, Oxford, pp 244–253

51. Levine MM, Kaper JB, Herrington D et al. (1988) Safety, immunogenicity and efficacy of recombinant live cholera vaccines. Lancet ii:467–470
52. Wicks ACB, Holmes GS, Davidson L (1971) Endemic typhoid fever. Q J Med 40:341–354
53. Cook GC (1980) Tropical gastroenterology. Oxford University Press, Oxford, pp 340–352
54. Mandal BK (1988) Typhoid fever and other salmonellae. Curr Opin Gastroenterol 4:1006–1009
55. Gupta SP, Gupta MS, Bhardwaj S, Chugh TD (1985) Current clinical patterns of typhoid fever. J Trop Med Hyg 88:377–381
56. Rose IN, Abraham T (1987) Predicting enteric fever without bacteriological culture results. Trans R Soc Trop Med 81:374–377
57. Archampong EQ (1985) Tropical disease of the small bowel. World J Surg 9:887–896
58. Christie AB (1971) Salmonellosis. Br J Hosp Med 5:331–340, 342
59. Mandal BK, Mani V (1976) Colonic involvement in salmonellosis. Lancet i:887–888
60. Day DW, Mandal BK, Morson BC (1978) The rectal biopsy appearances in *Salmonella* colitis. Histopathology 2:117–131
61. Asherkoff B, Bennett JV (1969) Effect of antibiotic therapy in acute salmonellosis on the fecal excretion of salmonellae. N Engl J Med 281:636–640
62. Cohen JI, Bartlett JA, Corey GR (1987) Extraintestinal manifestations of salmonella infections. Medicine 66:348–388
63. Cherubin CE, Kowalski J (1990) Non-typhoid *Salmonella* carrier state treated with norfloxacin. Ann Intern Med 85:100–101
64. Skirrow MB (1977) *Campylobacter* enteritis: a "new" disease. Br Med J ii:9–11
65. Lambert ME, Schofield PF, Ironside AG, Mandal BK (1979) *Campylobacter* colitis. Br Med J i:857–859
66. McNulty CAM (1987) The treatment of *Campylobacter* infections in man. J Antimicrob Chemother 19:281–284
67. Weir WRC (1985) *Campylobacter* infection. Curr Opin Gastroenterol 1:130–134
68. Levine MM (1987) *Escherichia coli* that cause diarrhoea: enterotoxigenic, enteropathogenic, enteroinvasive, enterohemorrhagic and enteroadherent. J Infect Dis 155:377–389
69. Riley LW, Remis RS, Helgerson SD et al. (1983) Hemorrhagic colitis associated with a rare *Escherichia coli* serogroup. N Engl J Med 308:681–685
70. Pai CH, Gordon R, Sims HV, Bryan LE (1984) Sporadic cases of hemorrhagic colitis associated with *Escherichia coli* 0157:H7: clinical, epidemiologic and bacteriologic features. Ann Intern Med 101:738–742
71. Carter AO, Borczyk AA, Carlson JAK et al. (1987) A severe outbreak of *Escherichia coli* 0157:H7 – associated hemorrhagic colitis in a nursing home. N Engl J Med 317:1496–1500
72. Goulston SM, McGovern VT (1965) Pseudomembranous colitis. Gut 6:207–211
73. Bartlett JG, Chang TW, Gurwith M, Gorbach SL, Onderdonk AB (1978) Antibiotic-associated pseudomembranous colitis due to toxin-producing clostridia. N Engl J Med 198:531–534
74. Gerding DN (1989) Disease associated with *Clostridium difficile* infection. Ann Intern Med 110:255–258
75. Bingley PJ, Harding GM (1987) *Clostridium difficile* colitis following treatment with metronidazole and vancomycin. Postgrad Med J 63:993–994
76. Roda PI (1987) *Clostridium difficile* colitis induced by cytarabine. Am J Clin Oncol 10:451–452
77. Testore GP, Pantosti A, Cerquetti M, Babudieri S, Panichi G, Mastrantonio Gianfrilli P (1988) Evidence for cross-infection in an outbreak of *Clostridium difficile*-associated diarrhoea in a surgical unit. J Med Microbiol 26:125–128
78. Larsen HE, Parry JB, Price AB, Davies DR, Dolby J, Tyrell DA (1977) Undescribed toxin in pseudomembranous colitis. Br Med J i:1246–1248
79. Price AB, Davies DR (1977) Pseudomembranous colitis. J Clin Pathol 30:1–12
80. Gebhard RL, Gerding DN (1988) *Clostridium difficile* disease. JAMA 259:3052
81. Bradley SJ, Weaver DW, Maxwell MPT, Bouwman DL (1988) Surgical management of pseudomembranous colitis. Am Surg 54:329–332
82. Thorne GM (1990) Diagnostic tests in gastrointestinal infections. Curr Opin Gastroenterol 6:79–88

83. Hromockyj AE, Maurelli AT (1989) Identification of *Shigella* invasion genes by isolation of temperature-regulated inv::lacz operon fusions. Infect Immunol 57:2963–2970
84. Speelman P, Kabier I, Islam M (1984) Distribution and spread of colonic lesions in shigellosis: a colonoscopic study. J Infect Dis 150:899–903
85. Panigrahi D, Agarwal KC, Verma AD, Dubey ML (1987) Incidence of shigellosis and multi-drug resistant shigellae: a 10-year study. J Trop Med Hyg 90:25–29
86. Cevallos AM, Farthing MJG (1991) Parasitic infections of the gastrointestinal tract. Curr Opin Gastroenterol 7:97–102
87. Weinke T, Freidrich-Jänicke B, Hopp P, Janitsche K (1990) Prevalence and clinical importance of *Entamoeba histolytica* in two high-risk groups: travellers returning from the tropics and male homosexuals. J Infect Dis 161:1029–1031
88. Allason-Jones E, Minder A, Sargeaunt P, Williams P (1986) *Entamoeba histolytica* as a commensal intestinal parasite in homosexual men. N Engl J Med 315:353–355
89. Vijrabukka T, Dhitarat A, Kichananta B et al. (1979) Fulminating amoebic colitis: a clinical evaluation. Br J Surg 66:630–632
90. Mtshali Z, Luvuno FM (1982) Progress in the management of amoebic colitis. Proceedings of the 13th biennial congress of the Association of Surgeons of South Africa, p 131
91. Luvuno FM (1990) Role of intraoperative prograde colonic lavage and a decompressive loop ileostomy in the management of transmural amoebic colitis. Br J Surg 77:156–159
92. Haddad FS, Ghossain A, Sawaya E, Nelson AR (1987) Abdominal tuberculosis. Dis Colon Rectum 30:724–735
93. Anand BS, Nanda R, Sachdev GK (1988) Response of tuberculous stricture to antituberculous treatment. Gut 29:62–69
94. Schofield PF (1985) Abdominal tuberculosis. Gut 26:1275–1278
95. Kasulke RJ, Anderson WJ, Gupta SK, Gliedman ML (1981) Primary tuberculous enterocolitis: report of three cases and review of the literature. Arch Surg 116:110–113
96. Jacubowski A, Elwood RK, Enarson DA (1987) Active abdominal tuberculosis in Canada in 1970–1981. Can Med Assoc J 137:897–902
97. Klimach OE, Ormerod LP (1985) Gastrointestinal tuberculosis: a retrospective review of 109 cases in a district general hospital. Q J Med 56:569–578
98. Schneebaum CW, Novick DM, Chabon AB et al. (1987) Terminal ileitis associated with *Mycobacterium avium-intracellulare* infection in a homosexual man with acquired immune deficiency syndrome. Gastroenterology 92:1127–1132
99. Gerberding JL (1989) Diagnosis and management of HIV-infected patients with diarrhoea. J Antimicrob Chemother 23(Suppl A):83–87.
100. Hoy J, Mitch A, Sandland M et al. (1990) Quadruple-drug therapy for *Mycobacterium avium-intracellulare* bacteremia in AIDS patients. J Infect Dis 161:801–805
101. Warren K (1983) Schistosomiasis. In: The Oxford textbook of medicine. D.J. Wetherall, J.G.G. Ledingham and D.A. Warrell (eds). Oxford University Press, Oxford, pp 449–455
102. De Cock KM (1986) Hepatosplenic schistosomiasis. A clinical review. Gut 27:734–745
103. Chapman PJC, Wilkinson PR, Davidson RN (1988) Acute schistosomiasis (Katayama fever) amongst British air crew. Br Med J 297:1101
104. Farid Z, Miner WF, Higashi GI, Hassan A (1976) Reversibility of lesions in schistosomiasis: a brief review. J Trop Med Hyg 79:164–166
105. Cook GC (1989) Parasitic infections of the gastrointestinal tract: a worldwide clinical problem. Curr Opin Gastroenterol 5:126–139
106. McMillan A, Lee FD (1981) Sigmoidoscopic and microscopic appearance of rectal mucosa in homosexual men. Gut 27:1035
107. Rodgers FG, Rodgers C, Shelton AP, Hawkey CJ (1986) Proposed pathogenic mechanism for the diarrhoea associated with human intestinal spirochetes. Am J Clin Pathol 86:679–682
108. Stürchler D (1987) Parasitic diseases of the small intestinal tract. Baillière Clin Gastroenterol 1:397–424
109. Anderson RM (1986) The population dynamics and epidemiology of intestinal nematode infection. Trans R Soc Trop Med 80:686–696
110. Louw JH (1966) Abdominal complications of *Ascaris lumbricoides* infection in children. Br J Surg 53:510–521
111. Turner JA (1986) Drug therapy of gastrointestinal parasitic infections. Am J Gastroenterol 81:1125–1137
112. Stephenson LS, Latham MC, Kurz KM, Kinoti SN, Brigham H (1989) Treatment with

a single dose of albendazole improves growth of Kenyan schoolchildren with hookworm, *Trichuris trichiuria* and *Ascaris lumbricoides* infections. Am J Trop Med Hyg 41:78–87
113. Wiersma R, Hadley GP (1988) Small bowel volvulus complicating intestinal ascariasis in children. Br J Surg 75:86–87
114. Mokoena T, Luvuno FM (1988) Conservative management of intestinal obstruction due to *Ascaris* worms in adult patients: a preliminary report. J R Coll Surg Edinb 33:318–321
115. Efem SE (1987) *Ascaris lumbricoides* and intestinal perforation. Br J Surg 74:643–644
116. Leung JWC, Chung SCS (1988) Endoscopic management of biliary ascariasis. Gastrointest Endosc 34:318–320
117. Cook GC (1986) The clinical significance of gastrointestinal helminths – a review. Trans R Soc Trop Med Hyg 80:675–685
118. Cook GC (1987) *Strongyloides stercoralis* hyperinfection syndrome. How often is it missed? Q J Med 64:625–630
119. Bundy DAP (1986) Epidemiological aspects of *Trichuris* and trichuriasis in Caribbean communities. Trans R Soc Trop Med Hyg 80:706–718
120. Forrester JE, Scott ME, Bundy DAP, Golden MNH (1988) Clustering of *Ascaris lumbricoides* and *Trichuris trichiuria* infections in households. Trans R Soc Trop Med Hyg 82:282–287
121. Nyberg W (1952) Microbiological investigation on antipernicious anemia factors in the fish tapeworm. Acta Med Scand S271:1–68
122. Richards F, Schantz PM (1985) Treatment of *Taenia solium* infections. Lancet i:1264–1265
123. Waki K, Oi H, Takahashi T, Nakabayashi T, Kitani T (1986) Successful treatment of *Diphyllobothrium latum* and *Taenia saginata* infection by intraduodenal gastrografin injection. Lancet ii:1124–1126
124. Gemmel MA (1988) Hydatid disease: a global health problem still to be solved. J Gastroenterol Hepatol 3:611–621
125. Marti-Bonmati L, Menor Serrano F (1990) Complication of hepatic hydatid cysts: ultrasound, computed tomography and magnetic resonance diagnosis. Gastrointest Radiol 15:119–125
126. Filice C, Diperri G, Strosselli M et al. (1990) Parasitologic findings in percutaneous drainage of human hydatid liver cysts. J Infect Dis 161:1290–1295

# 6 Inflammatory Bowel Disease

Wilks and Moxon (1875)[1] realised that there was an ulcerative condition of the colon which was non-infective. There was little progress in the management of ulcerative colitis over the next 59 years and in 1933, an article by Hardy and Bulmer[2], about the natural history of the disease, indicated that one third of their patients died within a year of onset of the disease.

The other non-specific inflammatory condition involving the large bowel is Crohn's disease. Dalziel (1913)[3] first described this granulomatous disease in the small bowel and the clinical and pathological features of small bowel disease were described by Crohn et al. (1932)[4]. Colp[5] in 1934 recognised that the colon could be involved in continuity. Lockhart-Mummery and Morson (1960, 1964)[6,7] indicated that the colon could be affected by Crohn's disease without ileal involvement. They described transmural inflammation and the presence of deep fissures as well as the presence of epithelioid granulomas in many, but not all, cases. Hawk et al. (1967)[8] gave a useful description of both the macroscopic and microscopic appearances in Crohn's disease.

It is only in the last 25 years or so that it has become recognised that both ulcerative colitis and Crohn's disease are causes of non-specific colonic inflammation and for this reason anything written about ulcerative colitis before 1970 has to be taken with some reservation (Mendeloff, 1975)[9]. Price (1978)[10] showed that although the distinction between colonic Crohn's disease and ulcerative colitis could be made in the majority of instances, there was a number in which it was difficult or impossible and he coined the term "colitis indeterminate" for these cases. It is accepted that about 10% of colitis cases fall into this group and the distinction is particularly difficult in acute fulminant colitis (Shepherd, 1991)[11]. The distinction is particularly important in patients who may have an ileoanal pouch constructed since it is believed that Crohn's disease is a contraindication to this operation (Beart, 1988)[12].

## Epidemiology and Aetiology

There have been many epidemiological reviews of inflammatory bowel disease in the last 20 years, each dealing with the disease in a particular geographical area. For this reason an overview is desirable and Sandler (1990)[13] reviews some of the recent papers on this subject and summarises the general conclusions. It is clear that inflammatory bowel disease has its highest incidence in Scandinavia, Great Britain and the United States though similar incidence occurs in some areas in Europe and Australasia. The reports from Asia and Africa indicate a very low incidence. There appears to be a slight female predominance in Crohn's disease and a slight male predominance in ulcerative colitis. Both diseases tend to show a bimodal age frequency with the first peak in the 20s and the second peak after 55. This latter is predominantly localised distal disease. There has been an increased incidence in the high-incidence areas until the last decade when the diseases appear to have plateaued. Much of the increased incidence has been due to an apparent increase in Crohn's disease from 1970. This may well be due to increased recognition. Whilst Crohn's disease and ulcerative colitis have many factors in common there are significant differences. Calkins (1989)[14] in a meta-analysis of previous studies showed that smoking was a protective factor with regard to the development of ulcerative colitis but increased the risk of developing Crohn's disease. Mucosal and immunological factors have been shown to differ between the two diseases (see later). In fact, Jenkins et al. (1990)[15] have suggested that ulcerative colitis should be considered to be two diseases because they find significant differences between localised distal disease and more extensive disease.

Psychiatric factors have been thought in the past to have aetiological importance but North et al. (1990)[16] reviewed all the English literature on the association between ulcerative colitis and psychiatric abnormality and demonstrated that all sound studies had failed to show such an association.

Roediger (1990)[17] reviewed studies which suggest that the colonic epithelium is functionally abnormal in ulcerative colitis. Podolsky and Fournier (1988)[18] have shown that patients with ulcerative colitis produced unique glycoproteins from their mucosa which are not produced in patients with Crohn's disease or in normal patients. Ramakrishna et al. (1991)[19] showed that patients with ulcerative colitis were unable to detoxify phenols in the colon whilst patients with Crohn's disease could do so. Further Gibson et al. (1988)[20] showed that cells of the colonic mucosa from ulcerative colitis patients were less able to retain $^{51}Cr$ than patients with Crohn's disease or normals. Hollander et al. (1986)[21] showed that patients with Crohn's disease and their healthy relatives had increased intestinal permeability to polyethylene glycol. This study has been expanded by Katz et al. (1989)[22] when they showed that patients with Crohn's disease had increased mucosal permeability to lactulose but their relatives had normal permeability to three oligosaccharides including lactulose. It is thought that this altered permeability may be important in the aetiology of Crohn's disease. There is no doubt that there is a marked increase in cytokines with enhanced activity of inflammatory mediators within the colonic wall in both types of inflammatory bowel disease. (Zipser, 1988)[23].

Vascular abnormalities in Crohn's disease were described by Thompson and Bowser (1980)[24]. Carr et al. (1986)[25] showed a markedly reduced vascular bed in patients with Crohn's disease. Wakefield et al. (1989)[26] further demonstrated the vascular pathology and highlighted the significance of local ischaemia in the pathogenesis.

There is no doubt that there is a strong family history in some patients with inflammatory bowel disease (IBD). Roth et al. (1989)[27] calculate that there is an 8.9% risk of IBD in children of patients and an 8.8% risk in siblings of patients. Farmer (1989)[28] reports an even higher incidence of familial disease. The genetic association is stronger in Crohn's disease than in ulcerative colitis.

Snook et al. (1989)[29] show that ulcerative colitis but not Crohn's disease has a significant association with accepted autoimmune diseases. Snook et al. (1991)[30] confirmed the presence of anticolonic antibodies in a minority of patients with ulcerative colitis. There are many local immunological reactions occurring in the bowel. These are well summarised by Zeitz (1990)[31] and Mahida (1990)[32]. Over the years there have been considerable efforts to implicate an infectious agent in Crohn's disease. Tanaka et al. (1991)[33] could find no evidence to support the involvement of any mycobacterium in Crohn's disease.

## Diagnosis

Clinical factors are important in distinguishing IBD from other types of colitis (Mandal, 1984)[34]. Schofield (1990)[35] summarises the clinical factors which frequently allow the clinician to distinguish Crohn's disease from ulcerative colitis. Bartholomeusz and Shearman (1989)[36] review the clinical and laboratory features helpful in assessing disease activity in Crohn's disease. Hodgson and Mazlam (1991)[37] discuss the various schemes for assessing disease activity in both ulcerative colitis and Crohn's disease with particular attention to their relevance in drug trials.

Lorusso et al. (1988)[38] confirm that whilst colonoscopy is the best method of assessing the extent of colonic involvement it may underestimate the extent of disease because biopsy of apparently normal mucosa may show histological evidence of inflammation. Potzi et al. (1989)[39] describe the different endoscopic appearances in Crohn's disease and ulcerative colitis. They stress the importance of biopsy from the edge of ulcers. Yao et al. (1989)[40] describe the mucosal abnormalities found in contrast studies of Crohn's disease. Balthazar and Chako (1990)[41] review the value of computed tomography (CT) in gastrointestinal disorders. It is beneficial in assessing complex fistulas and inflammatory masses. Koelbel et al. (1989)[42] suggest that magnetic resonance imaging (MRI) is a useful alternative to CT for similar indications. Crama-Bohbouth et al. (1988)[43] review the use of isotope-labelled granulocyte scans to assess the extent and severity of disease.

## Intestinal Complications

### Acute Toxic Dilatation

Gross dilatation of the colon in a "toxic" patient has been described in ulcerative colitis as evidence of severe life-threatening disease (Lumb et al., 1955)[44]. Smith et al. (1962)[45] suggested that both medication with codeine and barium enema in the acute phase tended to precipitate this complication. McInerney et al. (1962)[46] describe the clinical and radiological features. They emphasise the risk of perforation and the danger of the condition. Jalan et al. (1969)[47] set out the criteria for the diagnosis of toxic dilatation.

It has become realised that Crohn's colitis is subject to similar complications. Grieco et al. (1980)[48] found that the condition was commoner in Crohn's disease than in ulcerative colitis, whilst Greenstein et al. (1985)[49] report the reverse. Schofield et al. (1979)[50] describe toxic dilatation in infective colitis due to *Salmonella*. Subsequently, dilatation due to *Clostridium difficile* or other infective agents or ischaemia (Carr et al., 1986)[51] has been reported.

The treatment in non-infective states is emergency operation by ileostomy and colostomy (Turnbull et al., 1970)[52] or by colectomy (Goligher et al., 1970)[53].

Flatmark et al. (1975)[54] reported excellent results for subtotal colectomy, mucous fistula and ileostomy and this probably is the treatment of choice. Danovitch (1989)[55] stresses the need for early surgery in fulminant colitis and toxic dilatation and reviews the surgical techniques.

## Perforation

Free perforation in ulcerative colitis is usually associated with toxic dilatation (Edwards and Truelove, 1964)[56]. Schofield (1982)[57] reports that free perforation in Crohn's disease is rare but commoner than perforation in ulcerative colitis and is not usually preceded by dilatation of the colon.

Crohn's disease perforations may occur in both large and small bowel. Softley et al. (1988)[58] report a sharp fall in perforation associated with ulcerative colitis in recent years which they believe is due to prompter surgery in toxic patients.

## Psoas Abscess

Local abscess formation is common in Crohn's disease and it is now felt that Crohn's disease is amongst the commoner causes of psoas abscess (Leu et al. 1986)[59].

## Obstruction

Benign stricture formation in colitis is due to Crohn's disease in most cases but rarely produces obstruction (Morson, 1968)[60]. Many patients with small bowel Crohn's disease have symptoms due to incomplete obstruction but total obstruction is uncommon (Pennington et al., (1980)[61].

## Massive Haemorrhage

Edwards and Truelove (1964)[56] reported massive haemorrhage to be rare, occurring in less than 1% of ulcerative colitis patients. Greenstein et al.,

(1975)[62] noted that massive haemorrhage in colonic Crohn's disease, although rare, was commoner than in ulcerative colitis.

## Carcinoma and Dysplasia

Bargen (1928)[63] first reported carcinoma complicating ulcerative colitis. Slaney and Brooke (1959)[64] reported that the complication was rare before 10 years of disease and the risk increased as the length of history increased. Endling and Eklöf (1961)[65] showed the risk was much greater in total colitis than with limited disease. Patients with intermittently active disease have cancer risk similar to patients with continuous chronic disease (de Dombal et al., 1966)[66]. Kewenter et al. (1978)[67] state that patients with pancolitis of 10 years or more duration have a 20- to 30-fold risk of carcinoma and confirm that the risk is greatest in total or subtotal colitis. Recent papers (see p 95) suggest that the degree of risk had been somewhat exaggerated. Gyde et al. (1980)[68] have indicated that Crohn's disease of long standing also carries a high risk. In inflammatory bowel disease dysplasia in the epithelium of the large bowel is a histological marker for an increased risk of malignancy, as postulated by Warren and Sommers (1949)[69] in ulcerative colitis. Morson and Pang (1967)[70] demonstrated that dysplasia in ulcerative colitis is often widespread and can occur in flat, non-polypoid mucosa. They found in resected colons with carcinoma from patients with ulcerative colitis that there was almost inevitably patchy dysplasia. This was not only near the carcinoma but quite remote from it. This led to the suggestion of monitoring by rectal biopsy and subsequently by colonoscopy and multiple biopsies (Dickinson et al., 1980)[71]

Lennard-Jones et al. (1977)[72] analysed 229 patients who had undergone colonoscopy with biopsy. No patient had a carcinoma if biopsy did not show dysplasia and only 1 out of 20 patients with moderate dysplasia had a carcinoma but 4 of 7 patients with severe dysplasia who came to operation had a carcinoma.

Increased risk of carcinoma is not confined to ulcerative colitis and patients with Crohn's disease also have an increased risk (Weedon et al., 1973)[73]. Richards et al. (1989)[74] report 5 cases of carcinoma colon complicating Crohn's disease and all showed dysplasia. Korelitz et al. (1990)[75] show that rectal dysplasia is a marker for carcinoma in Crohn's disease. Riddell et al. (1983)[76] feel that once the dysplasia is identified in patients with ulcerative colitis, colectomy is the preferred treatment before waiting for the dysplasia to go to higher grade or to carcinoma-in-situ, but this is an extreme view. Filipe et al. (1985)[77] report that carcinoma can develop insidiously in the absence of dysplasia but this is rare. Jones et al. (1988)[78] confirm the increased incidence of carcinoma in ulcerative colitis and report that 2 asymptomatic carcinoma patients out of 3 showed high-grade dysplasia. It is now accepted that high-grade dysplasia should lead to advice for colectomy but low-grade dysplasia should be observed, in the absence of other signs (Lennard-Jones et al., 1990)[79]. Isbell and Levin (1989)[80] give an excellent review of colonoscopy, biopsy and dysplasia. In addition, they discuss biological markers of cellular perturbation that may precede dysplasia.

# Extraintestinal Complications

## Musculoskeletal

Wright and Watkinson (1965)[81] recorded that 45% of patients with ulcerative colitis had arthritis. This was usually fleeting and migratory. Less commonly there was ankylosing spondylitis and sacroiliitis. Janowitz and Sachar (1976)[82] show a similar incidence in Crohn's disease. Mallas et al. (1976)[83] record the high incidence of HLA-B27 histocompatibility antigen in these patients as evidence of genetic susceptibility to the disease. Many patients with arthritis also have ocular and cutaneous manifestations.

## Ocular

Edwards and Truelove (1964)[56] recorded the association of uveitis with ulcerative colitis in about 7% of their cases. Hopkins et al. (1974)[84] found a similar incidence in Crohn's disease. Coles (1982)[85] indicates that there are often joint or skin complications associated with uveitis.

## Cutaneous

Erythema nodosum occurs in about 2% of cases when the disease is active. It is often associated with arthritis. Pyoderma gangrenosum is a rare but serious complication (Edwards and Truelove, 1964)[56]. It may occur as an independent disease but about a third of cases are associated with inflammatory bowel disease (Thornton et al., 1980)[86].

## Hepatobiliary Disease

Gall stones are commoner in Crohn's disease (Heaton and Read, 1969)[87]. Minor liver disease is relatively common in both types of inflammatory bowel disease if the disease is severe. The most usual abnormality is fatty change (Eade et al., 1970)[88]. Pericholangitis is the other common finding and is non-progressive (Dordal et al., 1967)[89]. Cirrhosis is rare (Lupinetti et al., 1980)[90]. Nemeth et al. (1990)[91] confirmed these findings in children with inflammatory bowel disease. Sclerosing cholangitis and cholangiocarcinoma (Parker and Kendall, 1954)[92] occur with increased frequency in both types of IBD. Sclerosing cholangitis is associated with ulcerative colitis more commonly than with other diseases, including Crohn's disease (Chapman et al., 1980)[93]. Sclerosing cholangitis always involves both intrahepatic and extrahepatic elements (Thorpe et al., 1967)[94].

## Urinary Complications

These are of increased frequency in Crohn's disease. Schofield et al. (1968)[95] indicated that right ureteric stasis of a minor degree is common in Crohn's disease but manifest obstruction is rare. Present et al. (1968)[96] report right ureteric dilatation in almost 7% of patients with Crohn's disease. Ileovesical fistula complicates about 3% of patients with Crohn's disease (Kyle, 1980)[97]. There appears to be an increased incidence of urinary stones especially after colectomy for either ulcerative colitis or Crohn's disease and more commonly in ileal Crohn's disease than in ulcerative colitis (Deren et al., 1962)[98]. There is an increased incidence of amyloidosis with renal dysfunction in Crohn's disease (Lowdell et al., 1986)[99].

## Growth Retardation in Children

McCaffery et al. (1970)[100] highlighted the problems of growth restraint in IBD which can be such a disaster in children. Kirschner (1990)[101] reviews hormone studies on children with Crohn's disease and growth restraint. Barton and Ferguson (1990)[102] confirm that growth retardation occurs more frequently in Crohn's disease than ulcerative colitis. Davies et al. (1990)[103] indicate a growth spurt after successful surgery for Crohn's disease.

# Treatment

## Medical Management

Svartz (1942)[104] was the first to describe any effective treatment when she introduced sulphasalazine. Controlled therapeutic trials showed the value of this drug in ulcerative colitis (Baron et al., 1962)[105]. The American National co-operative Crohn's disease study (Summers et al., 1979)[106] and a multicentre European study (Malchow et al., 1984)[107] showed that oral sulphasalazine was better than placebo in colonic Crohn's disease in its initial effect but this effect was lost by 2 years. Misiewicz et al. (1965)[108] showed that maintenance with sulphasalazine markedly reduced the risk of relapse in inflammatory bowel disease. Azad Khan et al. (1977)[109] showed that the effective element in sulphasalazine was the salicylate moiety, 5-aminosalicylic acid (5-ASA) (mesalazine in Europe and mesalamine in the United States) whilst the sulphonamide was a carrier molecule with no therapeutic effect. However, the sulphonamide is responsible for the side-effects so other methods of carriage to the colon were explored. Meyers (1988)[110] reviews these new drugs and the assessment of the efficacy in trials. These drugs include pH-dependent resin or cellulose coating of ASA; azo-linkage of two molecules of ASA, olsalazine; or linkage of ASA to an inert carrier, balsalazine. They all have fewer side-effects than sulphasalazine and are equally effective. Laursen et al. (1990)[111] suggest that olsalazine gives higher concentrations of 5-ASA in the rectum than the other compounds.

It is possible to use 5-ASA rectally by enema or suppository. Biddle and Miner (1990)[112] report good long-term remission after treatment with mesalamine enemas. Campieri et al. (1990)[113] indicate that mesalazine suppositories are effective in inducing remission in distal proctitis.

Truelove and Witts (1955)[114] showed the effectiveness of systemic corticosteroids in a controlled trial and Truelove (1958)[115] showed that local steroids as retention enemas were effective in ulcerative proctitis. Truelove and Jewell (1974)[116] laid out a scheme for treatment of severe colitis including intravenous high-dose steroids coupled with surgery for deterioration or failure to improve, leading to a marked improvement in survival. Truelove (1988)[117] reviews medical management and whilst he continues to support steroids in the acute attack he cites compelling evidence to suggest that prolonged treatment with steroids is not indicated in ulcerative colitis. In both the American and European studies treatment with steroids shows a benefit in active Crohn's disease but not in quiescent disease.

Immunosuppressive treatment with azathioprine or its metabolite 6-mercaptopurine (6-MP) has been used as second-line treatment or as a steroid-sparing drug for more than 20 years in both ulcerative colitis and Crohn's disease. Present et al. (1980)[118] in a crossover trial showed that 6-MP was beneficial in Crohn's disease. Adler and Korelitz (1990)[119] showed the benefit of 6-MP on refractory ulcerative colitis. Lemann et al. (1990)[120] report on a 15-year experience with azathioprine with good response and maintenance rates in Crohn's disease. Allam et al. (1987)[121] reported a case of severe Crohn's disease in which intravenous cyclosporin A was able to produce significant improvement. Lightner and Present (1990)[122] reported on 15 patients with severe ulcerative colitis in which this new immunosuppressive drug was used. Eleven patients had responded within 8 days. Brynskov et al. (1989)[123] have carried out a multicentre double-blind trial of oral cyclosporin involving 71 patients. The group receiving the drug had a significantly better response rate than the placebo group.

Payne-James and Silk (1988)[124] review the situation of parenteral nutrition and conclude it is not a primary treatment for Crohn's disease. Greenberg et al. (1988)[125] indicate that simple enteral feeding helps symptomatic remission in Crohn's disease. O'Morain (1990)[126] reviews the role of nutrition and believes that enteral nutrition helps control acute attacks of Crohn's disease and is just as effective as parenteral nutrition. Allan (1988)[127], after reviewing the evidence, concludes that enteral or parenteral feeding may have a supporting role but there is little evidence that feeding plays any part in altering the natural history in Crohn's disease. He does not feel that there is compelling evidence that diet has a specific effect upon the disease or its progression.

Metronidazole may be helpful as an adjuvant in some situations. Bernstein et al. (1980)[128] demonstrated it was helpful in some cases of perineal Crohn's disease and Ursing et al. (1982)[129] suggested it was as effective as sulphasalazine in active Crohn's disease. Babb (1988)[130] reviews the use of metronidazole.

## Surgery: Ulcerative Colitis

Crile and Thomas (1951)[131] reported the use of total colectomy with ileostomy and described its clear advantage over ileostomy alone. Brooke (1952)[132] made an important contribution by describing the technique of eversion ileostomy which avoided previous problems of ileostomy maturation. Whilst proctocolectomy and ileostomy remained for many years the principal operation for ulcerative colitis, others proposed that most patients could be managed with a colectomy and ileorectal anastomosis. Aylett was the main proponent of this latter technique and reported favourable results (Aylett, 1960)[133]. The value of this type of restorative surgery was disputed by many surgeons including Goligher who reviewed the history of surgery in ulcerative colitis (Goligher, 1978)[134].

Kock (1969)[135] began to propose an operation with a reservoir at the end of the small bowel in an attempt to provide continence after total colectomy. His initial attempts were unsuccessful but in 1973 he proposed the designing of a non-return valve fashioned from the terminal ileum distal to the reservoir which did allow continence[136]. Parks and Nicholls (1978)[137] preserved the lower rectal musculature, the pelvic floor and the anal sphincters in an attempt to maintain continence after the construction of an S-shaped pouch which was anastomosed to the anal canal. Initially, many of the pouches had difficulty in emptying. As a result of this Utsunomiya et al. (1980)[138] described the formation of a U-shaped pouch which overcame the emptying difficulties. Nicholls (1987)[139] reviewed these two types of reservoir design and a four-limb W-pouch which he had previously proposed.

Dozois (1985)[140] gives a full account of the development of the surgical treatment of ulcerative colitis. Smith (1989)[141] compares the advantages, disadvantages and complications of the three options used as definitive treatment for ulcerative colitis, namely proctocolectomy with ileostomy, proctocolectomy with ileoanal pouch and colectomy with ileorectal anastomosis. Danovitch (1989)[142] lays down criteria for surgery in the acute case. If surgery is required in fulminant disease then ileostomy with colectomy but leaving the rectum is the treatment of choice as the initial operation.

Keighley and Kmiot (1990)[143] review the changes in the operation of ileoanal pouch but surgeons argue: should the pouch be stapled or sewn? (Curran and Hill, 1990)[144]; should the anastomosis be above the area of discrimination? (Johnston et al., 1987)[145]; should the pouch be J, S or W in shape? (Nicholls, 1987)[139]; and can the anus be everted safely? (Brough and Schofield, 1989)[146]. Smith and Orkin (1990)[147] make a valuable contribution in a review of the pathophysiology of the ileoanal pouch and continence. They point out how careful operative technique with respect for physiology can improve results.

## Surgery: Crohn's Disease

Crohn's disease activity indices (CDAI) have been postulated to assess the severity of disease (Best et al., 1976)[148]. Since Crohn's disease can involve any part of the gastrointestinal tract, anatomical localisation is important. Farmer et al. (1975)[149] proposed subdivision of Crohn's disease into ileal, ileocolic, colonic and miscellaneous. Manson and Schofield (1986)[150] felt that it was best to classify the common variants into predominantly ileal and predominantly colonic, omitting the ileocolic classification.

Oral ulceration may be aphthous but may have the characteristics of

Crohn's disease (Basu et al., 1975)[151]. Upper gastrointestinal Crohn's disease is rare but Nugent and Roy (1989)[152] have managed to review a large series. They find that many patients can be managed conservatively but if duodenal obstruction occurs, a gastroenterostomy without vagotomy is the treatment of choice.

Cohen (1989)[153] suggests that we should consider Crohn's disease, at whatever the presenting site, to be part of a patchy microscopic involvement of the whole of the gastrointestinal tract. Rutgeerts et al. (1990)[154] report on colonoscopy after ileal resection for Crohn's disease and find that there was biopsy evidence of Crohn's disease in the neoileum in 73% of patients within 1 year of operation but the majority of these patients are completely asymptomatic. A small group of patients were endoscoped 6 months after ileal resection and more than half had microscopic evidence of Crohn's disease despite negative biopsies from the residual ileum at the time of surgery. The so-called recurrence rate has been shown to be the same whether there is histological evidence of involvement at the resection margins or not (Pennington et al., 1980)[155]. These findings strongly support the contention that surgery in small bowel disease should be extremely conservative. Hultén (1988)[156] emphasises that this conservatism should be in the extent of resection but not in the willingness to undertake operation. He advocates early surgery in ileal disease, and stresses that any colonic resection should be minimal and that resections for recurrence should preserve large bowel. He records that if surgery is carried out before septic complications occur there is a highly significant lower postoperative complication rate as contrasted with patients in whom surgery is deferred until a complication occurs.

Alexander-Williams and Haynes (1985)[157] take us through the history of attempts at radical extensive resection, in continuity bypass and exclusion bypass. They emphasise the inferior results of these alternative procedures when compared with limited resection. Lee and Papaioannou (1982)[158] pioneered "minimal" surgery when they advocated short resections or stricturoplasty for suitable lesions. They adapted the idea from Katariya et al. (1977)[159] who reported a widening by longitudinal incision and transverse suture: stricturoplasty, used for tuberculous strictures. Alexander-Williams and Haynes (1985)[157] report from a centre where the senior author took an interest in stricturoplasty. They use this operation for recurrent and short multiple lesions but their usual treatment for primary ileal or ileocaecal Crohn's disease is resection. Dehn et al. (1989)[160] report the 10-year experience of the group who introduced stricturoplasty and showed it to be a safe procedure in selected patients with obstructive Crohn's disease due to a short, fibrous stricture. Whelan et al. (1989)[161] report that if there is no contamination, multiple anastomoses are as safe as single anastomosis, provided good technique is used.

Hill et al. (1988)[162] review external fistula complicating Crohn's disease. These may arise spontaneously, after drainage of an intraabdominal abscess or after definitive surgery for Crohn's disease. They lay down the principles of management with resuscitation and parenteral nutrition preceding investigation. Conservative treatment is advised for 6–8 weeks with control of sepsis. They recognise two types of fistula, those arising from undiseased bowel which may heal and those arising from involved bowel which do not heal and require later surgery for closure. The management of enterovesical fistula in Crohn's disease is reviewed by McNamara et al. (1990)[163].

Shivananda et al. (1989)[164] discuss recurrence and reoperation. They remind us of the difficulties of defining recurrence and point out that rates will differ depending on the criteria of recurrence. They recommend the use of second operation rate because that is the most objective criterion. They review other series and show that the second operation rate varies a little but in approximate terms it is 20% at 5 years, 35% at 10 years and 55% at 20 years after the first operation.

The other consequence of ileal resection is malabsorption with steatorrhoea which in the longer term is associated with gall stones and megaloblastic anaemia (Schofield, 1965)[165]. This study investigated vitamin $B_{12}$ absorption and showed that malabsorption occurred if more than 90 cm of ileum was excised but that it required some years before the anaemia became manifest. Andersson et al. (1978)[166] showed that terminal ileal resection led to bile salt malabsorption which induced diarrhoea and has proved to be the cause of the high incidence of gall stones previously observed.

Fazio (1986)[167] summarises the surgical options in colonic Crohn's disease; namely proctocolectomy and ileostomy when there is rectal and colonic disease; subtotal colectomy with anastomosis with a normal rectum and anal canal; segmental colectomy, and rarely the construction of an ileostomy for bowel rest. The principal dangers of rectal excision are disturbed sexual or urinary function (see pp 100–102) and poor healing of the perineal wound. Fazio emphasises that close rectal dissection can be used in IBD which will minimise autonomic nerve damage. Brough and Schofield (1991)[168] describe methods of dealing with the difficult perineal sinus problem.

Goligher (1985)[169] showed a recurrence rate of 20% at 12 years after proctocolectomy which is lower than after other excisions with anastomosis for Crohn's disease. His results for subtotal or total colectomy with ileosigmoid or ileorectal anastomosis (IRA) show a 71% recurrence in the neoileum on long-term follow-up despite strict criteria of rectal and anal normality before operation.

A malnourished patient or one with fulminant disease should be managed by subtotal colectomy and ileostomy. Harling et al. (1991)[170] report the results of this procedure and subsequent surgery. Rather less than one third of their patients have undergone IRA subsequently. If the rectum was severely diseased before operation then IRA was unlikely to be successful. Ambrose et al. (1984)[171] argue that despite the high recurrent operation rate after IRA the procedure is worthwhile as it gives several years without a stoma. Allan et al. (1989)[172] report satisfactory results after segmental colonic resection for isolated Crohn's lesions in the colon.

Gazzard (1987)[173] reviews various series that have attempted to analyse the quality of life as it is affected by Crohn's disease. He suggested that there is some evidence from the literature that surgical treatment may result in a better quality of life than medical treatment but feels that there is a need for newer and more objective measures to compare groups of patients in different ways.

# References


1. Wilks S, Moxon W (1875) Lectures on pathological anatomy, 2nd edn. Churchill, London
2. Hardy TL, Bulmer E (1933) Ulcerative colitis. Br Med J ii:812–815
3. Dalziel TK (1913) Chronic interstitial enteritis. Br Med J ii:1068–1070
4. Crohn BB, Ginzburg L, Oppenheimer GD (1932) Regional enteritis: a pathological and clinical entity. JAMA 99:1323–1329
5. Colp R (1934) A case of nonspecific granuloma of the terminal ileum and the cecum. Surg Clin North Am 14:443–449
6. Lockhart-Mummery HE, Morson BC (1960) Crohn's disease (regional enteritis) of the large intestine and its distinction from ulcerative colitis. Gut 1:87–105
7. Lockhart-Mummery HE, Morson BC (1964) Crohn's disease of the large intestine. Gut 5:493–509
8. Hawk WA, Turnbull RB, Farmer RG (1967) Regional enteritis of the colon. Distinctive features of the entity. JAMA 201:738–746
9. Mendeloff AI (1975) The epidemiology of idiopathic inflammatory bowel disease. In: Inflammatory bowel disease. J.B. Kirsner, R.G. Shorter (eds). Lea and Febiger, Philadelphia pp 3–19
10. Price AB (1978) Overlap in the spectrum of non-specific inflammatory bowel disease – colitis indeterminate. J Clin Pathol 31:567–577
11. Shepherd NA (1991) Pathological mimics of chronic inflammatory bowel disease. J Clin Pathol 44:726–733
12. Beart RW (1988) Proctocolitis and ileoanal anastomosis. World J Surg 12:160–163
13. Sandler RS (1990) The epidemiology of inflammatory bowel disease. Curr Opin Gastroenterol 6:531–535
14. Calkins BM (1989) A meta-analysis of the role of smoking in inflammatory bowel disease. Dig Dis Sci 34:1841–1854
15. Jenkins D, Goodall A, Scott BB (1990) Ulcerative colitis: one disease or two? (Quantitative histological differences between distal and extensive disease.) Gut 31:426–430
16. North CS, Clouse RE, Spitznagel EL, Alpers DH (1990) The relation of ulcerative colitis to psychiatric factors: a review of findings and methods. Am J Psychiatr 147:974–981
17. Roediger WEW (1990) The starved colon: diminished mucosal nutrition, diminished absorption and colitis. Dis Colon Rectum 33:858–862
18. Podolsky DK, Fournier DA (1988) Emergence of antigenic glycoprotein structures in ulcerative colitis detected through monoclonal antibodies. Gastroenterology 95:371–378
19. Ramakrishna BS, Roberts-Thompson IC, Pannall PR, Roediger WEW (1991) Impaired sulphation of phenol by the colonic mucosa in quiescent and active ulcerative colitis. Gut 33:46–49
20. Gibson PR, Van de Pol E, Barratt PJ, Doe WF (1988) Ulcerative colitis – a disease characterised by the abnormal colonic epithelial cell. Gut 29:516–521
21. Hollander D, Vadheim CM, Brettholz E, Petersen M, Delahunty T, Rotter JI (1986) Increased intestinal permeability in patients with Crohn's disease and their relatives. Ann Intern Med 105:883–885
22. Katz KD, Hollander D, Vadheim CM et al., (1989) Intestinal permeability in patients with Crohn's disease and their healthy relatives. Gastroenterology 97:927–931
23. Zipser RD (1988) Introduction: mediators of inflammation in inflammatory bowel disease. Dig Dis Sci 33 (Suppl):4S–5S
24. Thompson H, Bowser RS (1980) Granuloma, arteritis and inflammatory cell counts in Crohn's disease. In: Developments in gastroenterology: recent advances in Crohn's disease, vol 1. A.S. Pena et al. (eds). Martinus Nijhoff, Dordrecht, pp 80–83
25. Carr ND, Pullan BR, Schofield PF (1986) Microvascular studies in non-specific inflammatory bowel disease. Gut 27:542–549
26. Wakefield AJ, Sawyer AM, Dhillon AP et al. (1989) Pathogenesis of Crohn's disease: multifocal gastrointestinal infarction. Lancet ii:1057–1062
27. Roth MP, Petersen GM, McElree C, Feldman E, Rotter JI (1989) Familial empiric risk estimates of inflammatory bowel disease in Ashkenazi Jews. Gastroenterology 96:1016–1020
28. Farmer RC (1989) Study of family history among patients with inflammatory bowel disease. Scand J Gastroenterol 24 (Suppl 170):64–65

29. Snook JA, De Silva HJ, Jewell DP (1989) The association of autoimmune disorders with inflammatory bowel disease. Q J Med 72:835–840
30. Snook JA, Lowes JR, Wu KC, Priddle JD, Jewell DP (1991) Serum and tissue autoantibodies to colonic epithelium in ulcerative colitis. Gut 32:163–166
31. Zeitz M (1990) Immunoregulatory abnormalities in inflammatory bowel disease. Eur J Gastroenterol Hepatol 2:246–250
32. Mahida Y (1990) Macrophage function in inflammatory bowel disease. Eur J Gastroenterol Hepatol 2:251–255
33. Tanaka K, Wilks M, Coates PJ, Farthing MJG, Walker-Smith JA, Tabaqchali S (1991) *Mycobacterium paratuberculosis* in Crohn's disease. Gut 32:43–45
34. Mandal BK (1984) Differentiation of acute infective colitis and inflammatory bowel disease with coincident infection. Int Med Spec 3:175–190
35. Schofield PF (1990) Inflammatory disease of the large bowel. Surgery 85:2020–2026
36. Bartholomeusz FDL, Shearman DJC (1989) Measurement of activity in Crohn's disease. J Gastroenterol Hepatol 4:81–94
37. Hodgson HJF, Mazlam MZ (1991) Review article: assessment of drug therapy in inflammatory bowel disease. Aliment Pharmacol Therap 5:555–584
38. Lorusso D, Leo S, Dimatteo G, Giorgio P, Caruso ML (1988) Evaluation of the extent of ulcerative colitis: comparison between colonoscopic and histologic assessment. Coloproctology 4:212–214
39. Potzi R, Walfram M, Lochs H, Holzner H, Gangl A (1989) Diagnostic significance of endoscopic biopsy in Crohn's disease. Endoscopy 21:60–62
40. Yao T, Okada M, Fuchigami T et al. (1989) The relationship between the radiological and clinical features in patients with Crohn's disease. Clin Radiol 40:389–392
41. Balthazar EJ, Chako AC (1990) Computerized tomography in acute gastrointestinal disorders. Am J Gastroenterol 85:1445–1452
42. Koelbel G, Schmiedl U, Majer MC et al. (1989) Diagnosis of fistula and sinus tracts in patients with Crohn's disease: value of MR imaging. Am J Radiol 152:999–1003
43. Crama-Bohbouth GE, Arndt JW, Pena AS et al. (1988) Value of indium-III granulocyte scintigraphy in the assessment of Crohn's disease of the small intestine: prospective investigation. Digestion 40:227–236
44. Lumb G, Prothero RH, Ramsay GS (1955) Ulcerative colitis with dilatation of the colon. Br J Surg 43:182–188
45. Smith FW, Law DH, Nickel WF, Sleisenger MH (1962) Fulminant ulcerative colitis with toxic dilatation of the colon: medical and surgical management of 11 cases with observations regarding etiology. Gastroenterology 42:233–243
46. McInerney GT, Sauer WG, Baggenstoss AH et al. (1962) Fulminating ulcerative colitis with marked dilatation. Gastroenterology 42:244–257
47. Jalan KN, Sircus W, Card WI et al. (1969) An experience of ulcerative colitis. I. Toxic dilatation in 55 cases. Gastroenterology 57:68–82
48. Grieco MB, Bordan DC, Geiss AC, Beil AR (1980) Toxic megacolon complicating Crohn's disease. Ann Surg 191:75–80
49. Greenstein AJ, Sachar DB, Gibas A et al. (1985) Outcome of toxic dilatation in ulcerative and Crohn's colitis. J Clin Gastroenterol 7:137–143
50. Schofield PF, Mandal BK, Ironside AG (1979) Toxic dilatation of the colon in *Salmonella* colitis and inflammatory bowel disease. Br J Surg 66:5–9
51. Carr ND, Wells S, Haboubi NY et al. (1986) Ischaemic dilatation of the colon. Ann R Coll Surg Engl 68:264–266
52. Turnbull RB, Hawk WA, Schofield PF, Weakley F (1970) Choice of operation for the toxic megacolon phase of non-specific ulcerative colitis. Surg Clin North Am 50:1151–1169
53. Goligher JC, Hoffman DC, de Dombal FT (1970) Surgical treatment of severe attacks of ulcerative colitis with special reference to the advantages of early operation. Br Med J iv:703–706
54. Flatmark A, Fretheim G, Gjone E (1975) Early colectomy in severe ulcerative colitis. Scand J Gastroenterol 10:427–431
55. Danovitch SH (1989) Fulminant colitis and toxic megacolon. Gastroenterol Clin North Am 18:73–82
56. Edwards EC, Truelove SC (1964) The course and prognosis of ulcerative colitis. III. Complications. Gut 5:1–21
57. Schofield PF (1982) Toxic dilatation and perforation in inflammatory bowel disease. Ann R Coll Surg Engl 64:318–320

58. Softley A, Clamp SE, Bouchier IA et al. (1988) Perforation of the intestine in inflammatory bowel disease: an OMGE survey. Scand J Gastroenterol 23(Suppl 144):24–26
59. Leu S-Y, Leonard MB, Beart RW, Dozois RR (1986) Psoas abscess: changing patterns of diagnosis and etiology. Dis Colon Rectum 29:694–698
60. Morson BC (1968) Pathology. In: Ulcerative colitis. J.C.Goligher et al. (eds). Baillière Tindall and Cassell, London
61. Pennington L, Hamilton SR, Bayless TM et al. (1980) Surgical management of ulcerative colitis. Ann Surg 192:311–318
62. Greenstein AJ, Kark AE, Dreiling DA (1975) Crohn's disease of the colon. Am J Gastroenterol 6:40–48
63. Bargen JS (1928) Chronic ulcerative colitis associated with malignant disease. Arch Surg 17:561–576
64. Slaney G, Brooke BN (1959) Cancer in ulcerative colitis. Lancet ii:694–698
65. Endling NPG, Eklöf D (1961) Radiological findings and prognosis in ulcerative colitis. Acta Chir Scand 121:299–308
66. de Dombal FT, Watts J McK, Watkinson G, Goligher JC (1966) Local complications of ulcerative colitis: stricture, pseudopolyposis and carcinoma of the colon and rectum. Br Med J i:1442–1447
67. Kewenter J, Ahiman H, Hulten L (1978) Cancer risk in extensive ulcerative colitis. Ann Surg 188:824–828
68. Gyde SN, Prior P, Macartney JC et al. (1980) Malignancy in Crohn's disease. Gut 21:1024–1029
69. Warren S, Sommers CS (1949) Pathogenesis of ulcerative colitis. Am J Pathol 25:657–679
70. Morson BC, Pang LSC (1967) Rectal biopsies as an aid to cancer control in ulcerative colitis. Gut 8:423–434
71. Dickinson RJ, Dixon MF, Axon AT (1980) Colonoscopy and the detection of dysplasia in patients with longstanding ulcerative colitis. Lancet ii:620–622
72. Lennard-Jones JE, Morson BC, Ritchie JK, Shove DC, Williams CB (1977) Cancer in colitis: assessment of the individual risks by clinical and histological criteria. Gastroenterology 73:1280–1289
73. Weedon DD, Shorter RG, Ilstrup DM, Huizenga KA, Taylor WF (1973) Crohn's disease and cancer. N Engl J Med 289:1099–1103
74. Richards ME, Rickert RR, Nance FC (1989) Crohn's disease-associated carcinoma: a poorly recognised complication of inflammatory bowel disease. Ann Surg 209:764–773
75. Korelitz BI, Lauwers GY, Sommers SC (1990) Rectal mucosal dysplasia in Crohn's disease. Gut 31:1382–1386
76. Riddell R, Goldman H, Ransohoff DF et al. (1983) Dysplasia in inflammatory bowel disease: standardized classification with provisional clinical applications. Hum Pathol 14:931–968
77. Filipe MI, Edwards MR, Ehsanullah M (1985) A prospective study of dysplasia and carcinoma in the rectal biopsies and rectal stump of 8 patients following ileorectal anastomosis in ulcerative colitis. Histopathology 9:1139–1153
78. Jones HW, Grogono J, Hoare AM (1988) Surveillance in ulcerative colitis: burdens and benefits. Gut 29:325–331
79. Lennard-Jones JE, Melville DM, Morson BC, Ritchie JK, Williams CB (1990) Precancer and cancer in extensive ulcerative colitis: findings amongst 401 patients over 22 years. Gut 31:800–806
80. Isbell G, Levin B (1989) Ulcerative colitis and colonic cancer. Gastroenterol Clin North Am 17:773–791
81. Wright V, Watkinson G (1965) 1. The arthritis of ulcerative colitis. 2. Sacro-iliitis and ulcerative colitis. Br Med J ii:670–674, 675–680
82. Janowitz HD, Sachar DB (1976) New observations in Crohn's disease. Ann Rev Med 27:269–285
83. Mallas EG, Mackintosh P, Asquith P, Cook WT (1976) Histocompatability antigens in inflammatory bowel disease. Gut 17:906–910
84. Hopkins DJ, Horan E, Burton IL et al. (1974) Ocular disorders in a series of 332 patients with Crohn's disease. Br J Ophthalmol 58:732–737
85. Coles RS (1982) Implications of uveitis and other extra-intestinal manifestations in inflammatory bowel disease. B.I. Korelitz (ed). John Wright, Bristol, pp 15–19

86. Thornton JR, Teaque RH, Slow-Beer TS et al. (1980) Pyoderma gangrenosa and ulcerative colitis. Gut 21:247–248
87. Heaton KW, Read AE (1969) Gallstones in patients with disorders of the terminal ileum and distorted bile salt metabolism. Br Med J iii:494–496
88. Eade MN, Cooke WT, Brooke BN (1970) Liver disease in ulcerative colitis. Ann Intern Med 72:489–497
89. Dordal E, Glagov S, Kirsner JB (1967) Hepatic lesions in chronic inflammatory bowel disease. Gastroenterology 52:239–252
90. Lupinetti M, Mehigan D, Cameron JL (1980) Hepatobiliary complications of ulcerative colitis. Am J Surg 139:113–118
91. Nemeth A, Ejderhamn J, Glaumann H, Strandvik B (1990) Liver damage in juvenile inflammatory bowel disease. Liver 10:239–248
92. Parker RGF, Kendall EJC (1954) The liver in ulcerative colitis. Br Med J ii:1030–1032
93. Chapman RW, Marborough BA, Rhodes JM et al. (1980) Primary sclerosing cholangitis. Gut 21:870–877
94. Thorpe ME, Scheuer PJ, Sherlock S (1967) Primary sclerosing cholangitis: the biliary tree and ulcerative colitis. Gut 8:435–448
95. Schofield PF, Staff WG, Moore T (1968) Ureteral involvement in regional ileitis (Crohn's disease). J Urol 99:412–416
96. Present DH, Rabinowitz JG, Banks PA et al. (1968) Obstructive hydronephrosis. N Engl J Med 280:523–528
97. Kyle J (1980) Urinary complications of Crohn's disease. World J Surg 4:153–160
98. Deren JJ, Porush JG, Levitt MF et al. (1962) Nephrolithiasis as a complication of ulcerative colitis and regional enteritis. Ann Intern Med 56:843–853
99. Lowdell CP, Shousha S, Parkins RA (1986) The incidence of amyloidosis complicating inflammatory bowel disease. A prospective study of 177 patients. Dis Colon Rectum 29:351–354
100. McCaffery TD, Khosrow N, Lawrence AM, Kirsner JB (1970) Severe growth retardation in children with inflammatory bowel disease. J Pediatr 45:386–393
101. Kirschner BS (1990) Growth and development in chronic inflammatory bowel disease. Acta Paediatr Scand 366 (Suppl):98–104
102. Barton JR, Ferguson A (1990) Clinical features, morbidity and mortality of Scottish children with inflammatory bowel disease. Q J Med 277:423–439
103. Davies G, Evans CM, Shand WS, Walker-Smith JA (1990) Surgery for Crohn's disease in childhood: influence of disease and operative procedure on outcome. Br J Surg 77:891–894
104. Svartz N (1942) Salazopyrin, a new sulfanilamide preparation. Acta Med Scand 110:577–598
105. Baron JH, Connell AM, Lennard-Jones JE, Jones F (1962) Sulphasalazine and salicylazosulphadimidine in ulcerative colitis. Lancet i:1094–1096
106. Summers RW, Switz DM, Sessions JT Jr et al. (1979) National co-operative Crohn's disease study: results of drug treatment. Gastroenterology 77:847–869
107. Malchow H, Ewe K, Brandes JW et al. (1984) European co-operative Crohn's disease study: results of drug treatment. Gastroenterology 86:249–266
108. Misiewicz JJ, Lennard-Jones JE, Connell AM, Baron JH, Avery-Jones F (1965) Controlled trial of sulphasalazine in maintenance therapy for ulcerative colitis. Lancet i:185–188
109. Azad Khan AK, Piris J, Truelove SC (1977) An experiment to determine the active therapeutic moiety of sulphasalazine. Lancet ii:892–895
110. Meyers S (1988) The place of oral 5-aminosalicylic acid in the therapy of ulcerative colitis. Am J Gastroenterol 83:64–67
111. Laursen LS, Stokolm M, Bukhave K, Rask-Madsen J, Lauritsen K (1990) Disposition of 5-aminosalicylic acid by olsalazine and three mesalazine preparations in patients with ulcerative colitis: comparison of intraluminal colonic concentrations, serum values and urinary excretion. Gut 31:1271–1276
112. Biddle WL, Miner PB Jr (1990) Long-term use of mesalamine enemas to induce remission in ulcerative colitis. Gastroenterology 99:113–118
113. Campieri M, De Franchis R, Porro GB, Ranzi T, Brunetti G, Barbara L (1990) Mesalazine (5-aminosalicylic acid) suppositories in the treatment of ulcerative proctitis or distal proctosigmoiditis: a randomized controlled trial. Scand J Gastroenterol 25:663–668
114. Truelove SC, Witts LJ (1955) Cortisone in ulcerative colitis, final report on a therapeutic trial. Br Med J ii:1041–1048

115. Truelove SC (1958) Treatment of ulcerative colitis with topical hydrocortisone hemisuccinate sodium: a controlled trial employing restricted sequential analysis. Br Med J ii:1072–1077
116. Truelove SC, Jewell DP (1974) Intensive intravenous regimen for severe attacks of ulcerative colitis. Lancet i:1067–1070
117. Truelove SC (1988) Medical management of ulcerative colitis and indications for colectomy. World J Surg 12:142–147
118. Present DH, Korelitz BI, Wisch N, Glass JL, Sachar DB, Pasternack BD (1980) Treatment of Crohn's disease with 6-mercaptopurine. A long-term randomized, double-blind study. N Engl J Med 302:981–987
119. Adler DJ, Korelitz BI (1990) The therapeutic efficacy of 6-mercaptopurine in refractory ulcerative colitis. Am J Gastroenterol 85:717–722
120. Lemann M, Bonhomme P, Bitoun A, Messing B, Mogliani R, Rambaud JC (1990) Treatment of Crohn's disease with azathioprine or 6-mercaptopurine: retrospective study in 126 patients. Gastroenterol Clin Biol 14:548–554
121. Allam BF, Tillman JE, Thomson TJ, Crossling FT, Gilbert LM (1987) Effective intravenous cyclosporin therapy in a patient with severe Crohn's disease on parenteral nutrition. Gut 28:1166–1169
122. Lightner S, Present DH (1990) Preliminary report: cyclosporin in the treatment of severe active ulcerative colitis. Lancet 336:16–19.
123. Brynskov J, Freud L, Rasmussen SN et al. (1989) A placebo-controlled double-blind, randomized trial of cyclosporin therapy in active Crohn's disease. N Engl J Med 321:845–850
124. Payne-James JJ, Silk DB (1988) Total parenteral nutrition as primary treatment in Crohn's disease – RIP? Gut 29:1304–1308
125. Greenberg GR, Fleming CR, Jeejeebhoy KN, Rosenberg IH, Sales D, Tremaine WJ (1988) Controlled trial of bowel rest and nutritional support in the management of Crohn's disease. Gut 29:1309–1315
126. O'Morain CA (1990) Does nutritional therapy in inflammatory bowel disease have a primary or an adjunctive role? Scand J Gastroenterol 25 (Suppl 172):29–34
127. Allan RN (1988) Medical management: its accomplishments in Crohn's disease and indications for surgery. World J Surg 12:174–179
128. Bernstein LH, Frank MS, Brandt LJ, Boley SJ (1980) Healing of perianal Crohn's disease with metronidazole. Gastroenterology 79:357–365
129. Ursing B, Alm T, Baramy F et al. (1982) A comparative study of metronidazole and sulphasalazine for active Crohn's disease. Gastroenterology 83:550–562
130. Babb RR (1988) The use of metronidazole (Flagyl) in Crohn's disease. J Clin Gastroenterol 10:479–481
131. Crile G Jr, Thomas CY (1951) Treatment of acute toxic ulcerative colitis by ileostomy and simultaneous colectomy. Gastroenterology 19:58–68
132. Brooke BN (1952) The management of ileostomy. Lancet ii:102–104
133. Aylett SO (1960) Diffuse ulcerative colitis and its treatment by ileorectal anastomosis. Ann R Coll Surg Engl 27:260–284
134. Goligher JC (1978) The surgical treatment of colitis: past, present and future. Ann R Coll Surg Engl 60:258–260
135. Kock NG (1969) Intra-abdominal "reservoir" in patients with permanent ileostomy. Arch Surg 99:223–231
136. Kock NG (1973) Continent ileostomy. In: Progress in surgery. M. Allgower, S.E. Bergentz and R.Y. Carne (eds). Karger, Basle
137. Parks AG, Nicholls RJ (1978) Proctocolectomy without ileostomy for ulcerative colitis. Br Med J ii:85–88
138. Utsunomiya J, Iwama T, Imajo M, Matsuo S, Sawai S, Yalgashi K (1980) Total colectomy, mucosal proctocolectomy and ileo-anal anastomosis. Dis Colon Rectum 23:459–466
139. Nicholls RJ (1987) Restorative procto-colectomy with various types of reservoir. World J Surg 11:751–762
140. Dozois RR (1985) Alternatives to conventional ileostomy. Year Book, Chicago
141. Smith LE (1989) Surgical therapy in ulcerative colitis. Gastroenterol Clin North Am 18:99–110
142. Danovitch SH (1989) Fulminant colitis and toxic megacolon. Gastroenterol Clin North Am 18:73–82

143. Keighley MRB, Kmiot W (1990) Surgical options in ulcerative colitis: role of ileo-anal anastomosis. Aust NZ J Surg 60:835–848
144. Curran FT, Hill GL (1990) Results of 50 ileoanal J pouch operations. Aust NZ J Surg 60:579–583
145. Johnston D, Holdsworth PJ, Nasmyth DG et al. (1987) Preservation of the entire anal canal in conservative proctocolectomy for ulcerative colitis: a pilot study comparing end-to-end ileo-anal anastomosis without mucosal resection with mucosal proctectomy and endo-anal anastomosis. Br J Surg 74:940–944
146. Brough WA, Schofield PF (1989) An improved technique of J pouch construction and ileoanal anastomosis. Br J Surg 76:350–351
147. Smith LE, Orkin BA (1990) Physiology of the ileoanal anastomosis. Semin Colon Rect Surg 1:118–127
148. Best WR, Becktel JM, Singleton JW, Kern F (1976) Development of a Crohn's disease activity index. Gastroenterology 70:439–444
149. Farmer RG, Hawk WA, Turnbull RB (1975) Clinical patterns in Crohn's disease: a statistical study of 615 cases. Gastroenterology 68:627–635
150. Manson JM, Schofield PF (1986) Indications for and results of operation in inflammatory bowel disease. J R Soc Med 79:593–595
151. Basu MK, Asquith P, Thompson RA et al. (1975) Oral manifestations of Crohn's disease. Gut 16:249–254
152. Nugent FW, Roy MA (1989) Duodenal Crohn's disease: analysis of 89 cases. Am J Gastroenterol 84:249–254
153. Cohen Z (1989) Surgery in inflammatory bowel disease. Curr Opin Gastroenterol 5:514–519
154. Rutgeerts P, Geboes K, Ventrappen G, Beryls J, Kerremans R, Hiele M (1990) Predictability of the postoperative course of Crohn's disease. Gastroenterology 99:956–963
155. Pennington L, Hamilton SR, Bayless TM, Cameron JL (1980) Surgical management of Crohn's disease. Ann Surg 192:311–318
156. Hultén L (1988) Surgical treatment of Crohn's disease of the small bowel or ileocaecum. World J Surg 12: 180–185
157. Alexander-Williams J, Haynes IG (1985) Conservative operation for Crohn's disease of the small bowel. World J Surg 9:945–951
158. Lee ECG, Papaioannou N (1982) Minimal surgery for chronic obstruction in patients with extensive or universal Crohn's disease. Ann R Coll Surg Engl 64:229–233
159. Katariya RN, Sood G, Rao PG, Rao PL (1977) Stricturoplasty for tubercular stricture of the gastrointestinal tract. Br J Surg 64:496–498
160. Dehn TC, Kettlewell MG, Mortensen NJ, Lee ECG, Jewel DP (1989) Ten-year experience of stricturoplasty or resection for obstructive Crohn's disease. Br J Surg 76:339–341
161. Whelan RL, Wong WD, Goldberg SM, Rothenberger DA (1989) Synchronous bowel anastomoses. Dis Colon Rectum 32:365–368
162. Hill GL, Bourchier RG, Whitney GB (1988) Surgical and metabolic management of patients with external fistulas of the small intestine associated with Crohn's disease. World J Surg 12:191–197
163. McNamara MJ, Fazio VW, Lavery IC, Weakley FL, Farmer RG (1990) Surgical treatment of enterovesical fistulas in Crohn's disease. Dis Colon Rectum 33:271–276
164. Shivananda S, Hordijk ML, Pena AS, Mayberry JF (1989) Crohn's disease: risk of recurrence and reoperation in a defined population. Gut 30:990–995
165. Schofield PF (1965) The natural history and treatment of Crohn's disease. Ann R Coll Surg Engl 36:258–279
166. Andersson H, Filipson S, Hultén L (1978) Determination of the faecal excretion of labelled bile salts after intravenous administration of $^{14}$C-cholic acid. An evaluation of bile salt malabsorption before and after surgery in patients with Crohn's disease. Scand J Gastroenterol 13:249–255
167. Fazio VW (1986) Currently used surgical procedures for inflammatory bowel disease. In: Inflammatory bowel disease. F. T. de Dombal et al. (eds). Oxford University Press, Oxford, pp 523–578
168. Brough WA, Schofield PF (1991) The value of the rectus abdominis myocutaneous flap in the treatment of complex perineal fistula. Dis Colon Rectum 34:148–150
169. Goligher JC (1985) The long-term results of excisional surgery for primary and recurrent Crohn's disease of the large bowel. Dis Colon Rectum 28:51–55

170. Harling H, Hegnhøj J, Rasmussen TN, Jarnum S (1991) Fate of the rectum after colectomy and ileostomy for Crohn's disease. Dis Colon Rectum 34:931–935
171. Ambrose NS, Keighley MR, Alexander-Williams J, Allan RN (1984) Clinical impact of colectomy and ileorectal anastomosis in the management of Crohn's disease. Gut 25:223–227
172. Allan A, Andrews H, Hilton CJ, Keighley MRB, Allan RN, Alexander-Williams J (1989) Segmental colonic resection is an appropriate operation for short skip lesions due to Crohn's disease in the colon. World J Surg 13:611–616
173. Gazzard BG (1987) The quality of life in Crohn's disease. Gut 28:378–381

# 7 Small Bowel Ischaemia

Marston (1986)[1] reviews gut ischaemia which may be acute or chronic. It may be due to major or minor arterial blockage, venous occlusion or a low flow state. Wilson et al. (1987)[2] reviewed acute superior mesenteric ischaemia in 102 cases and found that 33% were due to embolus, 26% to thrombosis and 24% to low flow states. The condition was depressingly lethal with a survival of only 8%. They emphasise the difficulty in diagnosis because there are no specific clinical signs or laboratory tests which are diagnostic. Diagnosis is often made late and this makes the prognosis even worse. Treatment is by bowel resection with or without revascularisation. The revascularisation procedures of embolectomy, aortomesenteric shunt or endarterectomy are only applicable to the early case. Ottinger (1978)[3] reports that attempts at revascularisation often fail because of rethrombosis. Clavien (1990)[4] emphasises the importance of urgent selective superior mesenteric angiography (SMA) both to establish the nature and extent of the blockage and to give access for vasodilators or thrombolytic drugs. Boley et al. (1981)[5] report improved results in superior mesenteric artery vasodilatation with papaverine after revascularisation by embolectomy. Grendell and Ockner (1982)[6] showed that mesenteric venous occlusion has a better prognosis than other forms of infarction but that the recurrence rate is high. Clavien et al. (1989)[7] recommend contrast-enhanced computed tomography as the method of choice to demonstrate superior mesenteric vein thrombosis.

Assessment of bowel viability at operation in the early case can be difficult, whatever the cause. For this reason the use of Doppler ultrasound or flourescein and Wood's lamp may be of help in assessing the extent for resection (Mann et al., 1982)[8]. However, second-look laparotomy at 24 hours in the early case is still advocated by many (Lindblad and Hakansson, 1987)[9].

Chronic ischaemia involving the gut is due to occlusion or stenosis of at least two of the three major vessels supplying the gut and gives rise to intestinal angina, i.e. severe abdominal pain after eating, with steatorrhoea and weight loss (Mavor and Lyall, 1962)[10]. Marston et al.(1985)[11] give a retrospective review which emphasises the rarity of the condition when they report 22 cases suitable for vascular reconstruction in 22 years. Non-intrusive investigation by duplex Doppler scanning has good accuracy but aortography is still desirable before any attempt at surgical correction (Taylor, 1990)[12]. Baum et al. (1984)[13] described the surgical techniques of correction. Odurny et al. (1988)[14] describe successful percutaneous transluminal angioplasty in the treatment of intestinal angina.

Ischaemic intestinal injury may be due to medium or small vessel disease and has many underlying causes such as radiotherapy-induced enterocolitis or vasculitis of various causations. Lie (1987)[15] offered an excellent pathological classification of vasculitis. He defined vasculitis as inflammation of the blood vessels often accompanied by necrosis and occlusive changes. He classified vasculitis into three types according to the size of vessel. Large vessel disease includes Takayasu's disease and granulomatous giant cell arteritis. Medium-sized vessels are involved in polyarteritis nodosa and Wegener's granulomatosis. Vasculitis of small vessels occurs in hypersensitivity vasculitis, leucocytoclastic vasculitis, Henoch–Schonlein purpura and mixed cryoglobulinaemias. The clinical manifestations of vasculitis affecting the bowel relate very much to the size of the vessel involved, the location of the injury and the extent of the involvement. The pathological changes can vary from mucosal ulcers through deeper perforative ulceration to segmental transmural disease or necrosis. Stricture formation after recovery from more superficial damage may occur.

Luzar (1983)[16] states that the commonest forms of vasculitis affecting the gastrointestinal tract are polyarteritis nodosa and hypersensitivity angiitis. The gastrointestinal symptoms usually occur in the presence of systemic manifestation of the disease. Polyarteritis nodosa is characterised by inflammation and fibrinoid necrosis of small and medium-sized arteries with formation of microaneurysms. Immune complexes which may contain hepatitis B antigen are seen in up to 30% of patients. Cohen et al. (1980)[17] have shown that 25% of their patients with polyarteritis nodosa have gastrointestinal manifestations. In up to 15% of cases there are very severe complications such as gastrointestinal bleeding or abdominal pain progressing to segmental ischaemia and perforation. These more severe intestinal problems require surgical treatment.

Hypersensitivity vasculitis usually affects the skin, muscular tissue, kidney and the gastrointestinal tract (Lopez et al., 1980)[18]. Small vessels including small arteries, arterioles and capillaries are predominantly affected and sometimes the inflammation extends into the veins. Fibrinoid necrosis of the vessel wall and thrombosis are present together with a perivascular infiltrate of inflammatory cells, predominantly neutrophils. Similar changes are seen in Henoch–Schonlein purpura, cryoglobulinaemia and connective tissue disease associated vasculitis. In Henoch–Schonlein purpura, two thirds of the patients are under 16 years of age. Circulating IgA complexes are often demonstrated and IgA may be found deposited in the perivascular tissue. The disease usually affects the jejunum and ileum but can affect any part of the bowel (Lopez et al., 1980)[18]. The vascular changes lead to small haemorrhages, most commonly in the wall of the jejunum or ileum. Similar vascular changes are seen with cryoglobulinaemia but in this instance there are perivascular deposits of IgM. These changes lead to abdominal pain but this rarely requires any form of surgical treatment.

## References

1. Marston A (1986) Vascular disease of the gut: pathophysiology, recognition and management. Edward Arnold, Melbourne
2. Wilson C, Gupta R, Gilmour DG, Imrie CW (1987) Acute superior mesenteric ischaemia. Br J Surg 74:279–281

3. Ottinger LW (1978) The surgical management of acute occlusion of the superior mesenteric artery. Ann Surg 188:721–731
4. Clavien P-A (1990) Diagnosis and management of mesenteric infarction. Br J Surg 77:601–603
5. Boley SJ, Feinstein FR, Sammartano R, Brendt LJ, Sprayregen S (1981) New concept in the management of emboli of the superior mesenteric artery. Surg Gynecol Obstet 153:561–569
6. Grendell JH, Ockner RK (1982) Mesenteric venous thrombosis. Gastroenterology 82:358–372
7. Clavien P-A, Huber O, Mirescu D, Rohner A (1989) Contrast enhanced CT scan as diagnostic modality in mesenteric ischaemia due to mesenteric venous thrombosis. Br J Surg 76:93–94
8. Mann A, Fazio VW, Lucus FV (1982) A comparative study of the use of fluorescein and the Doppler device in the determination of intestinal viability. Surg Gynecol Obstet 154:53–55
9. Lindblad B, Hakansson H (1987) The rationale for "second-look operation" in mesenteric vessel occlusion with uncertain intestinal viability at primary surgery. Acta Clin Scand 153:531–534
10. Mavor GE, Lyall AD (1962) Superior mesenteric artery stenosis treated by iliac-mesenteric arterial bypass. Lancet ii:1143–1146
11. Marston A, Clarke JMF, Garcia S, Miller AL (1985) Intestinal function and intestinal blood supply: a 20-year surgical study. Gut 26:656–666
12. Taylor GA (1990) Blood flow in the superior mesenteric artery: estimated with Doppler ultrasound. Radiology 174:15–16
13. Baum GM, Millay DJ, Taylor LM Jr, Porter JM (1984) Treatment of chronic visceral ischemia. Am J Surg 148:138–144
14. Odurny A, Sniderman KW, Colapinto RF (1988) Intestinal angina: percutaneous transluminal angioplasty of the coeliac and superior mesenteric arteries. Radiology 167:59–62
15. Lie JT (1987) The classification and diagnosis of vasculitis in large and medium-sized blood vessels. In: Pathology annual, part 1. P.P. Rosen, R.E. Fechner (eds). Appleton-Century-Crofts, Norwalk, Connecticut, pp 125–162
16. Luzar MJ (1983) Systemic vasculitis. In: Intestinal ischaemia. M. Cooperman (ed). Futura, New York
17. Cohen RD, Corn DL, Ilstrup DM (1980) Clinical features, prognosis and response to treatment in polyarteritis. Proc Mayo Clinic 55:146–155
18. Lopez LR, Schocket AL, Stanford RE, Claman HN, Kohler PF (1980) Gastrointestinal involvement and leukocytic vasculitis and polyarteritis nodosa. J Haematol 7:677–684

# 8 Other Forms of Colitis and Enterocolitis

Shepherd (1991)[1] reviewed the histopathological appearances in a variety of colonic inflammatory conditions. He pointed out that these could be difficult to distinguish from ulcerative colitis or Crohn's disease and that there are many causes of inflammatory change within the colon which are not caused by acute infection, ulcerative colitis or Crohn's disease.

## Ischaemic Colitis

Boley et al. (1963)[2] in the United States and Marston et al. (1966)[3] in the United Kingdom pointed out that although major arterial blockage may well lead to complete infarction in some areas of the bowel, the colon was subject to a lesser ischaemic injury. In this, the vasa recta become blocked and necrosis of the mucosa, with or without some of the underlying muscle, may occur. This produces a typical syndrome of painful, bloody diarrhoea which may be self-limiting with return to normality or may go on to stricture formation. Boley et al. described the typical radiological appearance of thumbprinting on barium contrast studies. It was noted that the commonest site of injury was the splenic flexure. Griffiths (1956)[4] had shown that it was in this area that the colonic mesenteric anastomoses were at their most tenuous.

Smith and Szilagyi (1960)[5] described cases of left colonic ischaemia after aortic resection. Ernst (1983)[6] suggested that there was a postoperative incidence after aortic surgery of between 3% and 10%. West et al. (1980)[7] compared the minor self-limiting ischaemic colitis with the rarer total involvement of the colon. The more severe ischaemic injuries producing full-thickness necrosis may develop slowly and produce colonic dilatation (Carr et al., 1986)[8]. Far less commonly colonic ischaemia may be caused by venous occlusion (Wilson et al., 1987)[9]. This is suggested by the association of ischaemic colitis with contraceptive pill use in young women (Bétancourt et al., 1968)[10].

Ischaemic colitis can occur in the absence of vascular occlusion when it is associated with poor perfusion due to hypotension (Wilson and Qualheim, 1954)[11]. More recent animal experiments have shown that hypotension due to haemorrhage can produce localised or generalised colonic ischaemia (Matthews and Parks, 1976)[12]. The subject is well reviewed in Marston (1986)[13]. Necrosis due to poor perfusion is reviewed by Byrd et al., (1987)[14] who point out that the right colon tends to be the major colonic site of injury in this type of ischaemia.

Carr and Schofield (1982)[15] pointed out the difficulties for both the clinician and the histopathologist in distinguishing the long-term changes consequent upon prior ischaemia from the changes due to Crohn's disease. Morson et al. (1990)[16] discuss this difficulty and highlight the histopathological features indicative of an ischaemic aetiology.

## Diversion Colitis

Glotzer et al. (1981)[17] first noted that if the colon and/or rectum had the faecal stream diverted away from it, it may become inflamed and that this inflammation resolved when intestinal continuity was restored. Komorowski (1990)[18], reviewing the histopathology, noted that the condition could be difficult to distinguish from ulcerative colitis in some cases and that it could occur when the bowel had been defunctioned for non-inflammatory conditions such as tumour or incontinence.

It is suggested that the condition occurs due to inadequate nutrition of the mucosa (colonocytes). A review of this situation by Roediger (1990)[19] shows that the principal nutrient of the colonocyte is derived from short chain fatty acids, which are the principal anion in the lumen and responsible not only for nutrition but also for some elements of absorption. The short chain fatty acids are produced by the bacterial breakdown of carbohydrate, which either ceases or is much diminished when the bowel is defunctioned. Harig et al. (1989)[20] showed that perfusion of the defunctioned rectum with short chain fatty acids cured the diversion colitis and confirmed that diversion colitis was eliminated by reanastomosis. Geraghty and Talbot (1991)[21] confirm the histological spectrum and note that the patients may have no or minimal symptoms but do, on occasions, have bleeding or mucous discharge.

## Microscopic Colitis, Lymphocytic Colitis, Collagenous Colitis

Lindstrom (1976)[22] described a condition characterised by chronic watery diarrhoea but with minimal or no changes visible on colonoscopy or barium contrast studies. There was, however, abnormal histology on biopsy and he called this collagenous colitis due to the deposition of collagen in the subepithelial position. Kingham et al. (1982)[23] also described a chronic watery diarrhoeal state with normal investigations but abnormal pathology and they called this microscopic colitis. Sylwestrowicz et al. (1989)[24] feel that these two conditions should be grouped together. By contrast, Lazenby et al. (1989)[25] believe that distinctions should be made between the two conditions. They prefer to call microscopic colitis lymphocytic colitis because of the apparent intraepithelial lymphocyte infiltrate. Perri et al. (1989)[26] indicate that the diarrhoea may well be self-limiting or respond to sulphasalazine.

## Necrotising Enterocolitis

Whilst a variety of causes of intestinal necrosis and perforation have been recorded for many years in the medical literature it was not until the classical paper of Mizrahi et al. (1965)[27] that the entity of neonatal necrotising enterocolitis (NEC) was described from the clinical and radiological standpoint. The condition occurs more commonly in premature infants and in children on intensive care units. Wiswell et al. (1988)[28] estimate the incidence at 0.19 per 1000 live births. Despite improvements in management the condition still carries about a 30% mortality (Kleigman et al., 1982)[29]. Shanbhogue et al. (1991)[30] point to the danger of NEC developing in neonates of normal gestational age who undergo surgery in the neonatal period: 19% of their patients with NEC occurred after an operation and they believe that NEC must be in the differential diagnosis of any neonate who deteriorates during the period after any operation.

Although the radiology showing pneumatosis intestinalis and the pathology of patchy intestinal necrosis are characteristic of NEC the aetiology and pathogenesis are uncertain. The most widely accepted pathogenesis is that the condition is caused by ischaemia due to poor oxygenation associated with respiratory problems leading to anoxia (Bunton et al., 1977)[31]. Others have suggested that the primary basis is infective even suggesting *Clostridium difficile* as the organism (Han et al., 1983)[32] but subsequent work throws doubt upon this (Thomas et al., 1986)[33]. Others have suggested an association with *Clostridium perfringens* (Pedersen et al., 1976)[34]. This organism is known to cause enteritis in other circumstances and has been associated with the so-called pig-bel of New Guinea.

It seems probable that the causation is multifactorial. Eyal et al. (1982)[35] feel that the incidence can be reduced in premature infants if enteral feeding is delayed for 2–3 weeks after birth. The condition can often be managed medically by antibiotics and supportive therapy but surgery with resection and a temporary ileostomy is required if there are signs of perforation (Martin and Neblett, 1981)[36]. Kosloske (1985)[37] points to the importance of early recognition of gangrene before perforation, as operation at this stage halves the mortality. Resection for NEC is one of the major causes of short bowel syndrome and Caniano et al. (1989)[38] have indicated the much improved survival in recent years for infants with massive small bowel resection.

A similar necrotising enterocolitis may complicate the management of young children with Hirschsprung's disease and is the principal cause of death in this condition (Thomas et al., 1982)[39]. Archampong (1985)[40] discusses a necrotising enteritis seen in older children and young adults in Africa and compares it to "Darmbrand" described in Germany immediately after World War II and "pig-bel" in New Guinea. All these are lesions of the jejunum of uncertain causation.

## Neutropenic Colitis

Neutropenic colitis, also called the ileocaecal syndrome or typhilitis, was at first described in children with acute leukaemia or lymphoma undergoing chemotherapy. Varki et al. (1979)[41] reported it as a condition which previously had always been fatal and had usually been diagnosed at post mortem. It is now recognised that the condition can affect adults with haematological malignancy and more rarely with solid tumours (Keidan et al., 1989)[42].

Kunkel and Rosenthal (1986)[43] remark that the pathology does not show major vessel vascular occlusion but the terminal ileum, caecum and ascending colon are the subject of mucosal ulceration which may progress through intramural haemorrhage to necrosis and perforation. Clostridial infection, especially *C. septicum*, is believed to be the important causative factor by some authorities (King et al., 1984)[44]. Koea and Shaw (1989)[45] state that the cause is unknown but thrombocytopenia, low flow states and bacterial invasion of the mucosa may all be significant. These authors review the management and agree that at an early stage conservative management is appropriate but surgical intervention should not be withheld in a deteriorating situation. The appropriate treatment appears to be right hemicolectomy with terminal ileostomy and a mucous fistula (Vohra et al., 1992)[46].

## Radiation Enterocolitis

Therapeutic irradiation used in the treatment of malignant tumours may damage normal organs because effective dose fractionation regimes are near the tolerance of the surrounding normal tissues (Cox et al. 1986)[47]. Todd (1938)[48] indicated that radiotherapy for pelvic tumour was the most likely source of radiation injury and described an early acute phase and a more serious late phase. The early phase occurs in most patients during or shortly after pelvic irradiation whilst the late phase occurs in few patients, most commonly between 9 and 18 months after radiotherapy but may present many years later (Schofield et al., 1983)[49]. Injury can occur from intrauterine radionuclides or external beam radiotherapy and predominantly affects the pelvic colon and rectum or the small bowel. De Cosse et al. (1969)[50] review the small bowel injury and highlight the increased risk of radiation damage associated with previous pelvic surgery, hypertension or diabetes.

The pathology of the acute phase reaction has been little reported but Haboubi et al. (1988)[51] have described the changes at this phase which include nuclear changes with meganucleosis, eosinophilic infiltration into the mucosa and submucosal oedema. The histopathology of the late stage disease is better recognised and is well summarised by Berthrong (1986)[52]. Here the histopathological findings are focal ulceration in the mucosa with bizarre fibroblasts and abnormal vessels which may be telangiectatic, show microaneurysms or thrombosis. The full extent of the vascular changes at histopathology are emphasised by Hasleton et al. (1985)[53]. Carr et al.

(1984)[54] assessed the vascular changes in excision specimens by injection studies and showed a profound reduction in the microvascular volume and areas of necrosis in the bowel wall. These authors recognise that the changes may be quite widespread and emphasised that for successful surgery, relatively wide excision was necessary.

The late changes due to radiotherapy vary considerably in their severity from minor symptoms to major or even fatal illness. The usual clinical presentations may be rectal bleeding (Gilinsky et al., 1983)[55] partial or complete intestinal obstruction or rectovaginal fistula (Smith and De Cosse, 1986)[56]. Danielsson et al. (1991)[57] discuss the much rarer problem of chronic diarrhoea with malabsorption presenting some years after pelvic radiotherapy. Pilepich et al. (1983)[58] proposed a grading system for severity of radiation injury after treatment for carcinoma of the prostate and this has useful application to all radiation injury.

The minor degrees of injury can be managed conservatively (Zentler-Monroe and Bessel, 1987)[59]. There is no doubt that the more severe grades of radiation damage are difficult to treat. Smith and De Cosse (1986)[56] emphasise the importance of stabilising and correcting biochemical and metabolic deficiencies whilst investigating the patient and considering the role of surgery. A variety of operative scenarios have been proposed for rectal disease. It is still proposed by some that colostomy should be used as the first procedure or bypass in the case of small bowel disease (Wobbes et al., 1984)[60]. Most groups now appear to accept that excisional surgery with primary anastomosis is possible in many instances (Galland and Spencer, 1987)[61]. Detailed reviews of radiation-induced disease are contained in two recent monographs (Schofield and Lupton, 1989; Galland and Spencer, 1990)[62,63].

## Drug-Induced Enterocolitis

A number of drugs can induce small intestinal or colonic inflammation when taken by mouth. Non-steroidal anti-inflammatory drugs (NSAIDs) are probably the commonest cause of iatrogenic ileal and colonic ulceration and inflammation (Sheers and Williams, 1989)[64]. In the small bowel this may settle to produce multiple strictures. Gabriel et al. (1991)[65] have carried out a meta-analysis and shown that users of NSAIDS are at a three-fold greater risk of developing serious gastrointestinal problems than the general population. The risk is even greater in patients over the age of 60. Antineoplastic agents, especially 5-fluorouracil are a well-recognised cause of acute colitis (Floch and Hellman, 1965)[66]. Other well-known causes of acute colitis include methyl DOPA (Graham et al., 1981)[67] and gold (Jackson et al., 1986)[68]. Non-irritant rectal drugs or enemas cause little or no inflammation but rectal non-steroidals or irritant suppositories such as bisacodyl produce mild to moderate inflammatory changes (Levy and Gaspar, 1975)[69].

Small bowel problems are not only produced by NSAIDs but potassium-induced ulceration and strictures have been recognised for many years and were well reviewed by Boley et al. (1965)[70]. Oral contraceptive agents have been associated with acute ischaemia of the small bowel due to presumed venous occlusion (Hoyle et al., 1977)[71].

## Graft Versus Host Disease

Bone marrow transplantation for leukaemia is becoming an increasingly used therapy. Gastrointestinal symptoms are a common complication. The donor T cells react against the patient's cells in the liver, skin and intestine, producing jaundice, a macular or bullous rash and diarrhoea (McGregor et al., 1988)[72]. Sigmoidoscopy shows ulceration which is confirmed on histology (Spencer et al., 1986)[73]. Jones et al. (1988)[74] review the radiology which shows diffuse gastrointestinal changes which cannot be distinguished from viral enteritis (cytomegalovirus) by radiology alone. The condition is difficult to treat. It is fortunate that perforation is rare because surgery is unrewarding in this condition.

## References


1. Shepherd NA (1991) Pathological mimics of chronic inflammatory bowel disease. J Clin Pathol 44:726–733
2. Boley SJ, Schwartz S, Lash J, Sternhill V (1963) Reversible vascular occlusion of the colon. Surg Gynecol Obstet 116:53–60
3. Marston A, Pheils MT, Thomas ML, Morson BC (1966) Ischaemic colitis. Gut 7:1–10
4. Griffiths JD (1956) Surgical anatomy of the blood supply to the distal colon. Ann R Coll Surg Engl 19:241–256
5. Smith RE, Szilagyi DE (1960) Ischemia of the colon as a complication in the surgery of the abdominal aorta. Arch Surg 80:806–821
6. Ernst CB (1983) Prevention of intestinal ischaemia following abdominal aortic reconstruction. Surgery 93:102–106
7. West BR, Rae JE, Gathright JB (1980) Comparison of transient ischaemic colitis with that requiring surgical treatment. Surg Gynecol Obstet 151:366–368
8. Carr ND, Wells S, Haboubi NY, Salem RJ, Schofield PF (1986) Ischaemic dilatation of the colon. Ann R Coll Surg Engl 68:264–266.
9. Wilson C, Walker ID, Davidson JF, Imrie CW (1987) Mesenteric venous thrombosis and antithrombin III deficiency. J Clin Pathol 40:906–908
10. Bétancourt E, Farman J, Lawson JP (1968) Vascular occlusion of the colon and oral contraceptives. N Engl J Med 278:438–440
11. Wilson R, Qualheim RE (1954) A form of acute hemorrhagic enterocolitis afflicting chronically ill individuals. Gastroenterology 27:431–434
12. Matthews JGW, Parks TG (1976) Ischaemic colitis in the experimental animal. Gut 17:671–677
13. Marston A (1986) Vascular disease of the gut: pathophysiology, recognition and management. Edward Arnold, Melbourne, pp 152–173
14. Byrd RL, Cunningham MW, Goldman LI (1987) Non-occlusive ischaemic colitis secondary to hemorrhagic shock. Dis Colon Rectum 30:116–118
15. Carr ND, Schofield PF (1982) Inflammatory bowel disease in the older patient. Br J Surg 69:223–225
16. Morson BC, Dawson IMP, Day DW, Jass JR, Price AB, Williams GT (1990) Vascular disorders. In: Morson and Dawson's gastrointestinal pathology, 3rd edn. Blackwell Scientific, Oxford, pp 551–559.

17. Glotzer DJ, Glick ME, Goldman H (1981) Proctitis and colitis following diversion of the faecal stream. Gastroenterology 80:438–441
18. Komorowski RA (1990). Histologic spectrum of diversion colitis. Am J Surg Pathol 14:548–554
19. Roediger WEW (1990) The starved colon: diminished mucosal nutrition, diminished absorption and colitis. Dis Colon Rectum 33:858–862
20. Harig JM, Soergel KH, Komorowski RA, Wood CM (1989) Treatment of diversion colitis with short chain fatty acid irrigation. N Engl J Med 320:23–28
21. Geraghty JM, Talbot IC (1991) Diversion colitis: histological features in the colon and rectum after defunctioning colostomy. Gut 32:1020–1023
22. Lindstrom CG (1976) Collagenous colitis with watery diarrhoea: a new entity? Pathol Eur 11:87–89
23. Kingham JGC, Levison DA, Ball JA, Dawson AM (1982) Microscopic colitis: a cause of chronic watery diarrhoea. Br Med J 285:1601–1604
24. Sylwestrowicz T, Kelly JK, Hwang WS, Shaffer EA (1989) Collagenous colitis and microscopic colitis: the watery diarrhoea–colitis syndrome. Am J Gastroenterol 84:763–768
25. Lazenby A, Yardley J, Giardiello F, Jessurun J, Bayless T (1989) Lymphocyte ("microscopic") colitis. A comparative histopathologic study with particular reference to collagenous colitis. Hum Pathol 20:18–28
26. Perri F, Remotti D, Pescarmona E, Sarlo O (1989) Collagenous colitis: a clinicopathological review. Ital J Gastroenterol 21:286–292
27. Mizrahi A, Barlow O, Berdon W et al. (1965) Necrotizing enterocolitis in premature infants. J Pediatr 66:697–706
28. Wiswell TP, Robertson CF, Jones TA, Tuttle DJ (1988) Necrotizing enterocolitis in full-term infants: a case–control study. Am J Dis Child 142:532–535
29. Kleigman RM, Hack M, Jones P, Fanaroff AA (1982) Epidemiologic study of necrosing enterocolitis amongst low birthweight infants. J Paediatr 100:440–444
30. Shanbhogue LKR, Tam PKH, Lloyd DA (1991) Necrotising enterocolitis following operation in the neonatal period. Br J Surg 78:1045–1047
31. Bunton GL, Durbin GM, McIntosh N et al. (1977) Necrotising enterocolitis: controlled study of three years' experience in a neonatal intensive care unit. Arch Dis Child 52:772–777
32. Han VKM, Sayed H, Chance GW, Brabyn DG, Shaheed WA (1983). An outbreak of *Clostridium difficile* necrotizing enterocolitis: a case for oral vancomycin therapy? Pediatrics 71:935–941
33. Thomas DFM, Fernie DS, Bayston R, Spitz L, Nixon HH (1986) Enterocolitis in Hirschsprung's disease: a controlled study of the etiologic role of *Clostridium difficile*. J Pediatr Surg 21:22–25
34. Pedersen PV, Hansen FH, Halvez AB, Christiansen ED, Justensen T, Hgh P (1976) Necrotising enterocolitis of the newborn. Is it gas gangrene of the bowel? Lancet ii:715–716
35. Eyal F, Sagi E, Arad I, Avital A (1982) Necrotising enterocolitis in the very low birthweight infant: expressed breast milk feeding compared with parenteral feeding. Arch Dis Child 57:274–276
36. Martin LW, Neblett WW (1981) Early operation with intestinal diversion for necrotizing enterocolitis. J Pediatr Surg 16:252–255
37. Kosloske AM (1985) Surgery of necrotizing enterocolitis. World J Surg 9:277–284
38. Caniano DA, Starr J, Ginn-Pease ME (1989) Extensive short-bowel syndrome in neonates: outcome in the 1980s. Surgery 105:119–124
39. Thomas DFM, Malone M, Fernie DS, Bayston R, Spitz L (1982) Association between *Clostridium difficile* and enterocolitis in Hirschsprung's disease. Lancet i:78
40. Archampong EQ (1985) Tropical diseases of the small bowel. World J Surg 9:887–896
41. Varki AP, Armitage JO, Feagler JR (1979) Typhilitis in acute leukaemia. Cancer 43:695–697
42. Keidan RD, Fanning J, Gatenby RA, Weese JL (1989) Recurrent typhilitis: a disease resulting from aggressive chemotherapy. Dis Colon Rectum 32:206–209
43. Kunkel JM, Rosenthal D (1986) Management of the ileocaecal syndrome: neutropenic colitis. Dis Colon Rectum 29:196–199
44. King A, Rampling A, Wight DGP, Warren RE (1984) Neutropenic enterocolitis due to *Clostridium septicum* infection. J Clin Pathol 37:335–343

45. Koea JB, Shaw JHF (1989) Surgical management of neutropenic enterocolitis. Br J Surg 76:821–824
46. Vohra R, Prescott RJ, Banerjee SS, Wilkinson PM, Schofield PF (1992) Management of neutropenic colitis. Surg Oncol 1:11–15
47. Cox JD, Byhardt RW, Wilson JF, Haas JS, Komaki R, Olsen LE (1986) Complications of radiotherapy and factors in their prevention. World J Surg 10:171–188
48. Todd TF (1938) Rectal ulceration following irradiation treatment of carcinoma of the cervix uteri. Surg Gynecol Obstet 67:617–631
49. Schofield PF, Holden D, Carr ND (1983) Bowel disease after radiotherapy. J R Soc Med 76:463–466
50. De Cosse JJ, Rhodes RS, Wentz WB, Reagan JW, Dworken HJ, Holden WD (1969) The natural history and management of radiation-induced injury of the gastrointestinal tract. Ann Surg 170:369–384
51. Haboubi NY, Schofield PF, Rowlands P (1988) The light and electron microscopic features of early and late phase radiation-induced proctitis. Am J Gastroenterol 3:1140–1144
52. Berthrong M (1986) Pathologic changes secondary to radiation. World J Surg 10:155–170
53. Hasleton PS, Carr ND, Schofield PF (1985) Vascular changes in radiation bowel disease. Histopathology 9:517–534
54. Carr ND, Pullan BR, Hasleton PS, Schofield PF (1984) Microvascular studies in human radiation bowel disease. Gut 25:448–454
55. Gilinsky NH, Burns DG, Barbezat GO, Levin W, Myers HS, Marks IN (1983) The natural history of radiation induced proctosigmoiditis: analysis of 88 patients. Q J Med 52:40–53
56. Smith DH, De Cosse JJ (1986) Radiation damage to the small intestine. World J Surg 10:189–194
57. Danielsson A, Nyhlin H, Persson H, Stendahl U, Stenling R, Suhr O (1991) Chronic diarrhoea after radiotherapy for gynaecological cancer: occurrence and aetiology. Gut 32:1180–1187
58. Pilepich MV, Pajak T, George FW et al. (1983) Preliminary report on phase III RTOG studies of extended-field irradiation in carcinoma of the prostate. Am J Clin Oncol (CCT) 6:485–491
59. Zentler-Monroe PL, Bessel EM (1987) Medical management of radiation enteritis: an algorithmic guide. Clin Radiol 38:291–294
60. Wobbes T, Verschueren RC, Lubbers EJ, Janssen W, Paping RH (1984) Surgical aspects of radiation enteritis of the small bowel. Dis Colon Rectum 27:89–92
61. Galland RB, Spencer J (1987) Natural history and surgical management of radiation enteritis. Br J Surg 74:742–747
62. Schofield PF, Lupton EW (1989) The causation and clinical management of pelvic radiation disease. Springer, Berlin, Heidelberg, New York.
63. Galland RB, Spencer J (1990) Radiation enteritis, Edward Arnold, London
64. Sheers R, Williams WR (1989) NSAIDs and gut damage. Lancet ii:1154
65. Gabriel SE, Jaakkimainen L, Bombardier C (1991) Risk for serious gastrointestinal complications related to use of nonsteroidal anti-inflammatory drug: a meta-analysis. Ann Intern Med 115:787–796
66. Floch MH, Hellman L (1965) The effect of five-fluorouracil on rectal mucosa. Gastroenterology 48:430–437
67. Graham CF, Gallagher K, Jones JK (1981) Acute colitis with methyldopa. N Engl J Med 304:1044–1045
68. Jackson CW, Haboubi NY, Whorwell PJ, Schofield PF (1986) Gold-induced enterocolitis. Gut 27:452–456
69. Levy N, Gaspar E (1975) Rectal bleeding and indomethacin suppositories. Lancet i:577
70. Boley SJ, Schultz S, Kreiger H, Schwartz S, Elguezabal A, Allen AC (1965) Evaluation of thiazides and potassium as a cause of small bowel ulcer. JAMA 192:763–768
71. Hoyle M, Kennedy A, Prior AL, Thomas GE (1977) Small bowel ischaemia and infarction in young women taking oral contraceptives. Br J Surg 64:533–535
72. McGregor GI, Shepherd JD, Phillips GI (1988) Acute graft-versus-host disease of the intestine, a surgical perspective. Am J Surg 155:680–682
73. Spencer ED, Shulman HM, Myerson D et al. (1986) Diffuse intestinal ulceration after marrow transplantation: a clinical-pathologic study of 13 patients. Hum Pathol 17:621–633
74. Jones B, Kramer SS, Saral R et al. (1988) Gastrointestinal inflammation after bone marrow transplantation: graft-versus-host disease or opportunistic infection. AJR 150:277–282

# 9 Small Bowel Obstruction

McEntee et al. (1987)[1] review the causes of intestinal obstruction and show that in the UK and the USA external hernia was the commonest cause of small bowel obstruction (SBO) in the earlier part of the twentieth century, but recent series have shown a dramatic change with adhesions now the commonest cause of SBO in adults, though the exact frequency of these two causes varies widely. The increased number of adhesion obstructions has been attributed to the increased number of major abdominal operations. This is probably coupled with reduction in obstructed groin hernias due to early surgery for these conditions. McEntee et al. confirm that postoperative adhesions are the premier cause of SBO[1]. Ellis (1982)[2] notes this changing pattern of aetiology in the Western world but notes that obstructed external hernias still hold pride of place in the developing countries. He points out that most patients develop adhesions after operation but these are often protective; it is only in a minority of cases that obstruction occurs. He suggests that the reason for adhesion formation is minor local ischaemia. The two papers referred to indicate that extrinsic causes, whether adhesions or external hernia, are the cause of 80% of SBO. Sykes et al. (1973)[3] reported 81% of SBO to be due to extrinsic causes. They confirmed that femoral hernia carries the greater danger of obstruction and found that 40% of their patients presenting with obstructed femoral hernia required a resection as compared with 20% of the patients with an inguinal hernia. The remaining 19% of the series were described as obstruction without obvious cause. By this was meant that there was no cause which was apparent on clinical assessment. This latter group of patients were evenly spread between two subgroups, either with adherence to inflammatory intra-abdominal pathology such as diverticular disease, or intrinsic disease of the small bowel, either neoplasia or inflammatory bowel disease (Crohn's disease or tuberculosis).

Small bowel obstruction from incarceration in congenital intra-abdominal hernia is uncommon, accounting for less than 1% of small bowel obstruction. The specific diagnosis is rarely made preoperatively and may even be difficult at laparotomy as spontaneous reduction before or during surgery may occur. Hansmann and Morton (1939)[4] reviewed and classified the various types of internal hernia. Many of the hernias described by these authors occur through congenital defects caused by malfusion of peritoneum and mesentery although some are more likely to result from acquired peritoneal defects. Skandalakis and Gray (1987)[5] illustrate the variety of internal hernia which occurs around the duodenojejunal flexure, the ileocaecal region, through the diaphragm, through defects in the pelvis, the mesentery, the omentum, the broad ligament or the perineum. The radiological diagnosis of chronic reducible paraduodenal hernia causing intermittent symptoms was described by Meyers (1970)[6]. Passas et al. (1986)[7] and Day et al. (1988)[8] have emphasised the usefulness of computed tomography in the diagnosis of paraduodenal hernias when small bowel loops anterior to the pancreas indenting the posterior wall of the stomach may be demonstrated.

In all series, intraluminal obstruction proved to be rare, accounting for between 1% and 4% of cases. It may be due to gall stone ileus or food obstruction. Clavien et al. (1990)[9] give a very full review of gall stone ileus. Food obstruction is more common after gastrectomy or ileostomy and as many as 61 different foodstuffs have been incriminated (Stephens, 1966)[10]. There is an increasing list of rare iatrogenic causes: anticoagulants producing intramural haematoma (Herbert, 1968)[11], ileal stenosis after pelvic radiotherapy (Schmitt and Symmonds, 1981)[12], ulceration due to oral potassium (Leijonmarck and Räf, 1985)[13], ulceration due to non-steroidal anti-inflammatory drugs (Banerjee and Peters, 1990)[14] and intraluminal obstruction due to a foreign body, such as the "gastric bubble" used in the treatment of obesity (Zeman et al., 1988)[15].

In the neonate, the pattern of obstruction is totally different and is reviewed by Ricketts (1984)[16]. He states that obstruction is due to atresia in 80% of cases. In infants, obstructed hernia or intussusception are the common causes (Sykes et al., 1973)[3]. Agha (1986)[17] reviews intussusception and points out that only a small minority occurs in adults. In his series, 25 of 150 cases of intussusception were in adults. The principal cause was a benign or malignant tumour of the small bowel. The commonest age for intussusception in children is between 6 months and 3 years but at this stage there is no apparent tumour. It has been associated with viral infections particularly adenovirus (Gardner et al., 1962)[18]. It is suggested that this infection leads to hypertrophy of the Peyer's patches and these initiate the intussusception.

The other situation which requires special consideration is mechanical small bowel obstruction in the immediate postoperative period. Menzies and Ellis (1990)[19] show that 21% of adhesion obstructions occur within a month of operation and that this represents about 0.5% of cases submitted to laparotomy. Sykes and Schofield (1974)[20] analyse the clinical features and management. It is emphasised that the diagnosis is difficult and has to be distinguished from intestinal inhibition of non-mechanical nature – so-called paralytic or adynamic ileus. It should be recognised that after any type of abdominal surgery, normal upper gastrointestinal motility usually returns within 24 hours (Condon and Sarna, 1982)[21]. Sykes and Schofield (1974)[20] emphasise that whilst postoperative gastric and colonic dilatation are most commonly due to non-mechanical, self-limiting causes, small bowel dilatation is due to mechanical obstruction or significant sepsis or a combination of the two and is frequently an indication for reoperation. Quatromoni et al. (1980)[22] suggest that reoperation for obstruction carries about a 10% mortality but a lesser mortality is associated with intra-abdominal abscess.

The biggest danger in intestinal obstruction is that the obstructing factor may affect the blood supply to the segment of small bowel. This may produce simple engorgement due to venous obstruction or may produce arterial occlusion and infarction which may then progress to perforation. On this basis, Sarr et al. (1983)[23] suggested that small bowel obstruction should be divided into simple obstruction, viable strangulation and non-viable strangulation. They agreed with other groups that it was difficult or impossible to predict strangulation from clinical factors. Pain et al. (1987)[24] suggest that the diagnosis of strangulation may be assisted by the use of a computer. Others have accepted the difficulty of clinical differentiation and advocate immediate operation (Sykes et al., 1973; Davidson, 1981)[3,25]. The importance of strangulation is shown by the mortality rate after surgery. Bizer et al. (1981)[26] showed a 5.8% mortality in non-gangrenous small bowel obstruction whilst Barnett et al. (1976)[27] showed a mortality rate of 37% with strangulation obstruction.

Small bowel obstruction causes significant local and general changes. The bowel above the obstruction dilates with gas and then fluid. Most of the gas is nitrogen and appears to come from swallowed air (Chappuis and Cohn, 1987)[28]. Vomiting leads to fluid and electrolyte depletion which, if severe, has general haemodynamic effects (Billig and Jordan, 1969)[29]. The bacterial flora of the dilated bowel alters towards the colonic type with increased aerobes and colonisation with anaerobes (Sykes et al., 1976)[30]. The local vascular supply is increased and there is altered distribution to the mucosa and muscle layers of the bowel (Coxon and Taylor, 1987)[31]. In strangulation obstruction Ya et al. (1956)[32] showed that there was loss of blood from the circulation into the strangulated loop and if the loop was long this hypovolaemia could be fatal. However, there appear to be other factors which produce a more severe illness in strangulation. Cohn and Atik (1961)[33] showed that organisms proliferate and invade the devascularised bowel wall and produce a transudate of noxious fluid. Yale and Balish (1979)[34] showed that these ill effects did not occur in intestinal obstruction produced in germ-free dogs and conclude that the intestinal bacteria were a major lethal factor in strangulation. This may be due to exotoxins or endotoxin. The other factor which may be pertinent in strangulation obstruction is the risk of reperfusion injury which may lead to multisystem organ failure characterised by the adult respiratory distress syndrome, and renal, hepatic and cardiac insufficiency. Welbourn et al. (1991)[35] review the pathophysiology of reperfusion in which free oxygen radicals and arachnodonic acid products activate neutrophils which are disseminated and cause remote tissue injury.

Radiological investigations help to establish the diagnosis of small bowel obstruction. Simpson et al. (1985)[36] review the value of the plain film in the diagnosis and conclude that supine films alone are adequate for the diagnosis and that erect films may be omitted; a conclusion accepted by most radiologists but not by many clinicians. Beddi et al. (1985)[37] demonstrated that ultrasound can diagnose small bowel obstruction. Riveron et al. (1989)[38] discuss the use of contrast radiography in obstruction because they found that plain radiography alone was adequate for diagnosis in only 37% of patients. They found that useful information was obtained by contrast radiography in 86% of the remainder with little morbidity. Yuhasz et al. (1985)[39] found that small bowel enema was particularly valuable in assessing small bowel obstruction in patients who had previously undergone treatment for gynaecological malignancy. They state that obstruction in the upper small bowel was usually due to metastases whilst that in the lower small bowel was usually due to irradiation stricture. Dehn and Nolan (1989)[40] found small bowel enema useful in assessing patients with postoperative obstruction. In intussusception, barium enema is diagnostic and in children is usually effective in reducing the intussusception (Franken, 1988)[41].

Treatment of small bowel obstruction may be either conservative with nasogastric intubation and intravenous fluids or operative. A conservative policy is justified in incomplete obstruction since strangulation is virtually unknown and full investigation can be instituted (Bizer et al., 1981)[26]. The difficulty in predicting strangulation has led most surgeons to believe that early operation after rapid metabolic correction is the treatment of choice in most situations when the obstruction is complete (Davidson, 1981)[25].

The operative management is straightforward and depends on the cause of the small bowel obstruction. In general, the cause has to be eliminated and any non-viable bowel resected. Intraoperative Doppler ultrasound may help the assessment of viability (Cooperman et al., 1980)[42], and pulse oximetry has been shown to have an excellent discriminating power in distinguishing viable from non-viable bowel (De Nobile et al., 1990)[43]. Perioperative antibiotics are indicated and Krukowski et al. (1984)[44] show a minimal postoperative sepsis rate after peritoneal lavage with tetracycline in saline (1 g/l). Recurrent adhesion obstruction occurs in about 10% of patients after adhesiolysis and some of these patients go on to multiple episodes (Krook, 1947)[45]. In recurrent adhesion obstruction good results have been reported from the passage of a decompressing tube through the whole length of the small bowel and leaving it in situ for 2–3 weeks (Munro and Jones, 1978)[46]. Menzies and Ellis (1989)[47] have shown in experimental animals that tissue plasminogen activator prevents the formation of adhesions and this may become clinically practical in cases of recurrent adhesion obstruction.

## References


1. McEntee G, Pender D, Mulvin D et al. (1987) Current spectrum of intestinal obstruction. Br J Surg 74:976–980
2. Ellis H (1982) The causes and prevention of intestinal adhesions. Br J Surg 69:241–243.
3. Sykes PA, Grime RT, Schofield PF (1973) The management of small bowel obstruction. J R Coll Surg Edinb 18:169–175
4. Hansmann GH, Morton SA (1939) Intra-abdominal hernia: report of a case and review of literature. Arch Surg 39:973
5. Skandalakis JE, Gray SW (1987) Surgical anatomy of intestinal obstruction. In: Intestinal obstruction. L.P. Fielding, J.P. Welch (eds). Churchill Livingstone, Edinburgh, pp 14–31
6. Meyers MA (1970) Paraduodenal hernias. Radiologic and arteriographic diagnosis. Radiology 95:29–37
7. Passas V, Karavias D, Grilias D, Birbas A (1986) Computed tomography of left paraduodenal hernia. J Comput Assist Tomogr 10:542–543
8. Day DL, Drake DG, Leonard S, Letourneau JG (1988) CT findings in left paraduodenal herniae. Gastrointest Radiol 13:27–29
9. Clavien P-A, Richon J, Burgan S, Rohner A (1990) Gallstone ileus. Br J Surg 77:737–742
10. Stephens FO (1966) Intestinal colic caused by food. Gut 7:581–582
11. Herbert DC (1968) Anticoagulant therapy and acute abdomen. Br J Surg 55:353–357
12. Schmitt EH, Symmonds RE (1981) Surgical treatment of radiation-induced injuries of the intestine. Surg Gynecol Obstet 153:896–900
13. Leijonmarck CE, Räf L (1985) Ulceration of the small intestine due to slow-release potassium chloride tablets. Acta Surg Scand 151:273–278
14. Banerjee AK, Peters TJ (1990) Crohn's disease and NSAID enteropathy: a unifying model. Gastroenterology 99:1190–1191

15. Zeman RK, Benjamin SB, Cunningham MB et al. (1988) Small bowel obstruction due to Garren gastric bubble: radiographic diagnosis. AJR 150:581–582
16. Ricketts RR (1984) Workup of neonatal intestinal obstruction. Am Surg 50:517–521
17. Agha FP (1986) Intussusception in adults. Review. AJR 146:527–731
18. Gardner PS, Knox EG, Court SDM, Green CA (1962) Virus infection and intussusception in childhood. Br Med J ii:697–700
19. Menzies D, Ellis H (1990) Intestinal obstruction from adhesions: how big is the problem? Ann R Coll Surg Engl 72:60–63
20. Sykes PA, Schofield PF (1974) Early postoperative small bowel obstruction. Br J Surg 61:594–600
21. Condon RE, Sarna SK (1982) Motility after abdominal surgery. Clin Gastroenterol 11:609–620
22. Quatromoni JC, Rosolf L, Halls J, Yellin AE (1980) Early postoperative small bowel obstruction. Ann Surg 191:72–74
23. Sarr MG, Bulkley GB, Zuidema GD (1983) Preoperative recognition of intestinal strangulation obstruction. Am J Surg 145:176–182
24. Pain JA, Collier D St J, Hanka R (1987) Small bowel obstruction: computer-assisted prediction of strangulation at presentation. Br J Surg 74:181–183
25. Davidson AJ (1981) Early operation in the treatment of small bowel obstruction. J Natl Med Assoc 73:245–246
26. Bizer LS, Liebling RW, Delaney HM, Gliedman ML (1981) Small bowel obstruction. The role of non-operative treatment in simple intestinal obstruction and predictive criteria for strangulation obstruction. Surgery 89:407–413
27. Barnett WO, Petro AB, Williamson JW (1976) A current appraisal of problems with gangrenous bowel. Ann Surg 183:653–659
28. Chappuis CW, Cohn I (1987) Pathophysiological effects on intraluminal contents. In: Intestinal obstruction. L.P. Fielding, J.P. Welch (eds). Churchill Livingstone, Edinburgh, pp 32–40
29. Billig DM, Jordan PH (1969) Hemodynamic abnormalities in intestinal obstruction. Surg Gynecol Obstet 128:1274–1282
30. Sykes PA, Boulter KH, Schofield PF (1976) The microflora of the obstructed bowel. Br J Surg 63:521–525
31. Coxon JE, Taylor I (1987) Blood flow and peristalsis. In: Intestinal obstruction. L.P. Fielding, J.P. Welch (eds). Churchill Livingstone, Edinburgh, pp 41–48
32. Ya PM, Perry JF, Thein MS, Wangensteen OH (1956) Measurement of sequestration of red cell mass in strangulating intestinal obstruction utilizing radioactive $^{51}$Cr. Surg Forum 7:411–415
33. Cohn I, Atik M (1961) Strangulation obstruction in closed loop studies. Ann Surg 153:94–102.
34. Yale CE, Balish E (1979) Intestinal strangulation in germ-free and monocontaminated dogs. Arch Surg 114:445–448
35. Welbourn CRB, Goldman E, Paterson IS, Valeri CR, Shepro D, Hechtman HB (1991) Pathophysiology of ischaemia reperfusion injury: central role of the neutrophil. Br J Surg 78:651–655
36. Simpson A, Sandeman D, Nixon SJ, Goulbourne IA, Grieve DC, MacIntyre IMC (1985) The value of an erect abdominal radiograph in the diagnosis of intestinal obstruction. Clin Radiol 86:41–42
37. Beddi BG, Fagan CJ, Nocera M (1985) Sonographic diagnosis of bowel obstruction presenting with fluid-filled loops of bowel. J Clin Ultrasound 13:23–30
38. Riveron FA, Obeid FN, Horst HM, Sorensen VJ, Bivins BA (1989) The role of contrast radiography in presumed bowel obstruction. Surgery 106:496–501
39. Yuhasz M, Laufer I, Sutton G, Herlinger H, Caroline DF (1985) Radiography of the small bowel in patients with gynecological malignancies. AJR 144:303–307
40. Dehn TCB, Nolan DJ (1989) Enteroclysis in the diagnosis of intestinal obstruction in the early postoperative period. Gastrointest Radiol 14:15–21
41. Franken EA (1988) Non-surgical treatment of intussusception. AJR 150:1353–1354
42. Cooperman M, Martin EW, Carey LC (1980) Evaluation of ischaemic intestine by Doppler ultrasound. Am J Surg 139:73–77
43. De Nobile J, Guzzetta P, Patterson K (1990) Pulse oximetry as a means of assessing bowel viability. J Surg Res 48:21–23

44. Krukowski ZH, Stewart MP, Alsayer HM, Matheson NA (1984) Infection after abdominal surgery: five-year prospective study. Br Med J 288:278–280
45. Krook SS (1947) Obstruction of the small intestine due to adhesions and bands. Acta Surg Scand 95 (Suppl 125):1–200
46. Munro A, Jones PF (1978) Operative intubation in the treatment of complicated small bowel obstruction. Br J Surg 65:123–127
47. Menzies D, Ellis H (1989) Intra-abdominal adhesions and their prevention by topical tissue plasminogen activator. J R Soc Med 82:534–535

# 10 Tumours of the Small Intestine

It is not easy to subdivide tumours into benign and malignant categories in all cases. However, Olmsted et al. (1987)[1] review those tumours which have little or no malignant predisposition. These tumours are often asymptomatic and are less common than malignant small bowel tumours. The common varieties are the lipoma, the leiomyoma and the adenoma. However, Olmsted excludes the latter two groups as they have a definite malignant potential. He does include Peutz–Jeghers polyps which now also appear to have malignant potential (Spigelman et al., 1989)[2]. The other tumours highlighted in Olmsted's series are the neural tumours associated with neurofibromatosis, "adenoma" of Brunner's glands and fibroid polyps. If benign tumours produce symptoms, they do so either due to causing an intussusception or by bleeding due to ulceration of the mucosa overlying them.

Weiss and Yang (1987)[3] carried out an epidemiological study of malignant tumours of the small intestine. Their data came from several cancer registries in the United States reporting cases in the decade up to 1982. They state that there is an annual incidence of malignant small bowel tumours of 9.6 per million population, composed of 3.9 adenocarcinomas, 2.9 carcinoid tumours, 1.6 lymphomas and 1.2 sarcomas. Carcinomas occur more commonly in the duodenum and are less common in the jejunum and least common in the ileum. Carcinoid tumours and lymphomas are most common in the ileum whilst sarcomas have an even distribution. Taggart and Imrie (1987)[4], investigating cases seen in the previous 25 years, conclude that the histological pattern is changing and that lymphomas have become the predominant small bowel tumour.

## Investigation

Johnson et al. (1985)[5] indicated the diagnostic difficulty in small bowel tumours which may present as obscure abdominal pain or bleeding but often do not present until they undergo the complication of obstruction or perforation. Brophy and Kahow (1989)[6] found that 64% of patients with small bowel tumours presented as surgical emergencies.

The available investigations include barium contrast studies, computed tomography, angiography and endoscopy. Maglinte and Herlinger (1989)[7] review the difficulties in barium contrast studies and conclude that small bowel enema (enteroclysis) is much the most accurate contrast method with a diagnostic accuracy of over 90% for small bowel tumours. Computed tomography is seen as an adjunct to contrast radiography. Tillotson et al. (1988)[8] review mesenteric angiography in patients with small bowel bleeding. If a lesion is found from which contrast is not extravasated one third of the patients were found to have a neoplasm. Upper gastrointestinal endoscopy is useful in the diagnosis of adenomas and adenocarcinomas since a majority of these are present in the duodenum. Many of these are associated with familial adenomatous polyposis (Van Stolk et al., 1987)[9]. Lewis and Waye (1988)[10] reviewed small bowel enteroscopy for gastrointestinal bleeding in which a small bore long enteroscope is allowed to pass to the caecum spontaneously over several hours. Examination of the whole small bowel is carried out as it is withdrawn. In this review of 60 patients they discovered that 20 had vascular malformations but only one patient had a small bowel tumour.

## Adenocarcinoma

Adenocarcinomas of the small intestine have been reported as complications of the hereditary polyposis syndromes: familial adenomatous polyposis (FAP) (Van Stolk et al., 1987)[9]; Peutz–Jeghers polyposis (Spigelman et al., 1989)[2] and juvenile polyposis (Bentley et al., 1989)[11]. Richards et al. (1989)[12] report further examples of small bowel adenocarcinoma complicating Crohn's disease whilst coeliac disease which has a very strong association with lymphoma appears to have a less pronounced but positive association with adenocarcinoma (Fishman et al., 1990)[13].

## Neuroendocrine Tumours

Tumours may arise from cells in the APUD system. These tumours may affect a single organ or multiple organs. In the gut the enterochromaffin cells may give rise to tumours which contain and/or secrete hormones. The symptoms may be local but may be due to the secretion if it is in excess of the body's ability to degrade it. The tumours are rare and in the gut the usual tumour contains 5-hydroxytryptamine (5-HT) and is described as a carcinoid tumour (Walter and Israel, 1979)[14].

These neoplasms can arise anywhere in the gastrointestinal tract and have been classified into foregut, mid-gut and hindgut categories based on the embryological derivation of their site of origin (William and Sandler 1963)[15]. Foregut carcinoids have a trabecular or mixed architectural pattern. Gastric carcinoids are often microadenomas or endocrine cell hyperplasia (Moertel et al., 1961)[16]. They are usually non-argentaffin in type. Most carcinoids arise in the mid-gut, especially the appendix and the distal ileum. Mid-gut carcinoids are usually of argentaffin type, i.e. they exhibit silver staining which demonstrates intracellular granules which consist of 5-HT. They also show a strong argyrophilia whilst hindgut carcinoids show argyrophilia only (Willander et al., 1977)[17]. Marks (1979)[18] indicated that mid-gut carcinoids were multicentric in 40% of cases. He also noted that mid-gut carcinoids were often associated with primary malignant neoplasms at other sites.

It is difficult to predict tumour behaviour from microscopic appearances. It has now become clear that all carcinoids are potentially malignant and that the tendency for aggressive behaviour is related to the anatomical site, the extent of intramural penetration by the tumour cells and the size of the tumour (Marks, 1979)[18]. Appendicular carcinoids show malignant behaviour in less than 1% of cases and metastasis in rectal carcinoids is uncommon (Sanders, 1973)[19]. Carcinoids of the terminal ileum are more aggressive than those in the rest of the gastrointestinal tract. More than two thirds of the tumours greater than 2 cm in diameter show metastasis when first discovered while those under 1 cm in size show metastasis in less than 5% of cases (Morgan et al., 1974)[20].

Creutzfeldt and Stöckmann (1987)[21] give an excellent review of carcinoids and the carcinoid syndrome. They note that less than 10% of patients with carcinoid have the carcinoid syndrome. They describe the carcinoid syndrome as occurring in patients with liver metastases, most commonly from a mid-gut carcinoid. The syndrome consists of flushing of the face and neck, diarrhoea, bronchospasm and thickening of the endocardium of the right heart leading to tricuspid or pulmonary stenosis. The syndrome is associated with excess 5-HT and kallikrein. Recognition of the breakdown product of 5-HT, 5-hydroxyindole-acetic acid, in the urine, is used as a confirmatory test. Norheim et al. (1987)[22] analyse hormone production and show that in the carcinoid syndrome high levels of other hormones may be detected. More rarely the carcinoid syndrome is associated with foregut carcinoids when the excess hormones appear to be principally 5-HT and histamine which produce a particularly severe variant. Grahame-Smith (1987)[23] has published several articles on the carcinoid syndrome over the years. He recognises four types of flush in carcinoids but is still not able to be certain of the chemical factors responsible for the flush though 5-HT acting synergistically with bradykinin produced from kallikrein seems to be important. The diarrhoea is due to 5-HT.

Woods et al. (1985)[24] lay down the aims of treatment in carcinoid, namely to remove the primary tumour radically if it is still localised. If it is widespread the aim is to reduce the tumour mass by resection of the primary tumour and secondary deposits within the abdomen and liver. They review the place of hepatic artery ligation or embolisation in the treatment of liver secondaries. Bukowski et al. (1987)[25] reviewed cytotoxic therapy which was shown to be of little value. Recently the use of a somatostatin analogue has been shown to control symptoms (Souquet et al., 1987)[26]. Interferon appears to have growth restraining ability. Norheim et al. (1987)[22] indicate that a combination of interferon and a somatostatin analogue gives benefit in terms of survival as well as symptomatic improvement.

Tumours of the enterochromaffin cells are responsible for a group of rare syndromes.

## The Gastrinoma Syndrome (Zollinger–Ellison Syndrome)

In 1955 Zollinger and Ellison[27] described a condition characterised by ulceration of the small intestine associated with tumours of the pancreas. Later it was shown that gastrin is the active principal peptide responsible for the syndrome. The gastrin secretion by the neoplasm stimulates the acid-secreting cells of the body of the stomach to maximal activity with consequent liability to duodenal or jejunal ulceration (Walsh and Grossman, 1975)[28]. At least 50% of these tumours are malignant. Most of the tumours arise in the islet cells of the pancreas but up to 10% may arise in the duodenum, mostly in the second part (Oberhelman, 1972)[29]. Sometimes gastrinomas of the stomach are multiple and have occasionally been seen to arise on a background of pre-existing antral G cell hyperplasia.

The diagnosis of the Zollinger–Ellison syndrome depends upon the demonstration of a significantly elevated basal serum gastrin level; the demonstration of a paradoxical increase in serum gastrin levels after secretin stimulation; the finding of pancreatic or extrapancreatic tumours; the demonstration of very high gastrin levels in the venous effluent from the tumour preoperatively or intraoperatively (Walsh and Grossman, 1975)[28].

## Vipoma (Verner–Morrison Syndrome)

This is most usually associated with a pancreatic tumour but can occur with an intestinal tumour. It is characterised by watery diarrhoea, hypokalaemia and achlorhydria and has been called the WDHA syndrome (Soergel, 1975)[30].

## Somatostatinoma Syndrome

This is typically characterised by diabetes mellitus, diarrhoea, steatorrhoea, hypochlorhydia or achlorhydria, weight loss and anaemia (Gander et al., 1977)[31]. Most of the tumours are of pancreatic origin and only a handful have been described in the intestine. Most tumours are malignant and have a high incidence of metastasis.

## Cushing's Syndrome

Whereas adrenocorticotrophic hormone (ACTH) production can be frequently demonstrated in gastrointestinal carcinoid, it is rare for such ectopic ACTH production to cause clinical manifestations of Cushing's syndrome (Marcus et al., 1980)[32]. In these rare cases the tumour has arisen from foregut-derived structures such as lung or stomach. Mostly the tumours were malignant with metastasis to the regional lymph nodes (Herata et al., 1976)[33].

## Multiple Endocrine Neoplasm Syndromes (MEN)

Given the widespread distribution of the neuroendocrine cells it is not surprising that there should be cases where there are neoplasms at multiple sites. There are two rare syndromes which are well recognised. Both are familial and are inherited as a dominant (Welbourn, 1977)[34]. MEN type I or Wermer's syndrome includes parathyroid adenomas and may include islet cell tumours of the pancreas or gastrinoma or vipoma or other tumours of the enterochromaffin system. MEN II or Sipple's syndrome has as its main features hyperparathyroidism with medullary carcinoma of the thyroid, phaeochromocytoma and possibly other abnormalities of neuroectodermal origin.

# Gastrointestinal Lymphoma

Extranodal lymphoma is uncommon, but the gastrointestinal tract is a frequent location for this type of disease (Freeman et al., 1972)[35]. It should be emphasised that the term gastrointestinal lymphoma is reserved for disease involving the wall of the gut with or without lymph node involvement but should not be used for abdominal disease affecting only the lymph nodes. Lymphomatous involvement of the gut may be primary or secondary. Wright and Isaacson (1983)[36] defined primary intestinal lymphoma as "those presenting in the gastrointestinal tract necessitating the direction of diagnostic investigation and treatment to that site". Almost all primary intestinal lymphomas are of the non-Hodgkin's type (Lewin et al., 1978)[37]. By contrast, secondary lymphoma occurs when there is involvement of the gut late in advanced disease, after the patient has presented with lymphoma at other sites. Secondary involvement of the gut is found in approximately 40% of non-Hodgkin's lymphoma and in approximately 20% of Hodgkin's lymphoma at autopsy (Cornes, 1967)[38]. The type, distribution and location of lymphomas is different in the West from that seen in Middle Eastern countries. Wright and Isaacson (1989)[39] offer a classification of primary intestinal lymphomas into B cell lymphoma arising in mucosa-associated lymphoid tissue (Western type and Eastern type); Burkitt's and Burkitt-like lymphoma; multiple lymphomatous polyposis; enteropathy associated T cell lymphoma; and Mediterranean lymphoma (immunoproliferative small intestinal disease (IPSID)). Hall et al. (1988)[40] suggest a slightly different classification:

*B cell*

| | | |
|---|---|---|
| Low grade | Polymorphic small B cell | Aozasa et al. (1988)[41] |
| | IPSID: Third World type | Khojasteh et al. (1983)[42] |
| | Western type | Matuchansky et al. (1988)[43] |
| | Multiple lymphomatous polyposis | Blackshaw (1980)[44] |
| High grade | Polymorphic large B cell | Aozasa et al. (1988)[41] |
| | Burkitt-type | Anaissie et al. (1985)[45] |

| *T cell* | | |
|---|---|---|
| Low grade | Sporadic | Kanavaros et al. (1988)[46] |
| High grade | Enteropathy associated | Isaacson et al. (1985)[47] |

In developed countries localised lymphoma is the common type, whilst in the Middle East, primary small bowel lymphoma represents 50% of all extranodal disease and a majority of patients have IPSID (Al-Bahrani et al., 1983)[48]. For this reason the clinical presentation is different in developed countries and the Middle East.

### *Western B Cell Lymphoma*

In Western countries, presentation is usually with insidious onset of abdominal pain and vomiting and possibly altered bowel habit but some patients present as an emergency with perforation, obstruction or major bleeding (Green et al., 1979)[49]. Baildam et al. (1989)[50] note that the diagnosis is often delayed because of the ill-defined nature of the symptoms and the presumption of a more common disease such as peptic ulcer in gastroduodenal lymphoma or Crohn's disease when there is ileal involvement. Both these series and others show that gastroduodenal disease is the commonest site followed by ileal disease, with a colonic site of disease being relatively infrequent. Endoscopy with biopsy may make the diagnosis but can be misleading (Baildam et al., 1989)[50]. Small bowel contrast studies may suggest the diagnosis of small bowel lymphoma but it is difficult to distinguish from Crohn's disease and computed tomography may well be used to complement barium studies (Siegal et al., 1988)[51]. In order completely to stage the disease, chest radiography and bone marrow aspiration are required but a laparotomy with resection of localised disease is necessary for histological diagnosis.

Grody et al. (1985)[52] showed that the majority of Western gastrointestinal lymphomas were of B cell origin. Aozasa et al. (1988)[41] described the distribution and histology of gastrointestinal lymphoma and felt that the most significant prognostic factor was the histological classification of the tumour. They also confirmed that pleomorphic small cell tumours had a better prognosis than large cell tumours. They noted that gastric lymphoma appeared to have a better prognosis than small intestinal lymphoma and suggested that it should be considered separately. Hockey et al. (1987)[53] reviewed 153 patients with primary gastric lymphoma and reported that 97% were non-Hodgkin's lymphoma. They suggested that surgery is the more satisfactory treatment and report a 66% resectability rate with an age-adjusted 5-year survival rate of 24%. However, if the lesion was less than 5 cm in size the survival is reported as 63% but with poor survival in stages III and IV disease. They do not find that adjuvant radiotherapy or radiotherapy as a primary treatment in early disease can be substantiated. Perrin and Blackledge (1986)[54] report disappointing results with chemotherapy in gastrointestinal lymphoma when compared with the results seen in nodal disease.

Zwigler (1984)[55] shows that there is a definite increase in the incidence of non-Hodgkin's lymphoma in patients with acquired immunodeficiency disease syndrome (AIDS). The distribution along the gastrointestinal tract is similar to the pleomorphic B cell lymphoma but in the AIDS patients the lymphoma is highly aggressive (Joachim et al., 1985)[56]. The result of treatment in this situation is extremely poor with a life expectancy of less than 1 year (Kaplan et al., 1987)[57] Patients who have long-term immunosuppression, in particular survivors in transplant programmes, have an increased risk of lymphoma (Hoover and Fraumeni, 1973)[58].

## Immunoproliferative Small Intestinal Disease (IPSID)

The presentation in patients from the Middle East is usually that of malabsorption with severe weight loss, finger clubbing and abdominal pain (Al-Bahrani et al., 1983)[48]. IPSID involves long sections of the small bowel, in particular the duodenum and proximal jejunum. Characteristically there is an abnormal alpha chain circulating in the serum and found in the duodenal juice (Al-Bahrani et al., 1983)[48]. The histological basis of IPSID is a diffuse plasmocytic or lymphoblastic infiltrate involving a long segment of the upper small intestine which gradually changes into frank lymphoma. Three stages of IPSID have been described (Galian et al., 1977)[59]. Stage A is where the plasmocytic infiltrate is confined to the mucosa expanding the villi and compressing the crypts. The lymph nodes may contain excess plasma cells. It is at this stage that they may respond to treatment with broad-spectrum antibiotics producing remission or cure. Stage B is when there is transformation to lymphoma. The cellular infiltrate extends below the muscularis mucosa and lymphoid nodules appear in the mucosa with atypical lymphocytes or plasma cells. Stage C is marked by the presence of a frank tumour mass or masses but spread beyond the gastrointestinal tract is a late phenomenon. The epithelial infiltrate is by parafollicular B cells (Wright and Isaacson, 1983)[36]. As in the Western B cell lymphoma there are lymphoepithelial lesions so that both can be categorised as tumours of the mucosa-associated lymphoid tissue (MALT) or gastrointestinal-associated lymphoid tissue (GALT). Smith et al. (1987)[60] have shown that clonal immunoglobulin gene rearrangements occur in Stage A IPSID, i.e. the premalignant stage. They suggest that the plasma cell infiltrate in IPSID appears to be monoclonal in origin and depends on non-specific antigenic drive produced by luminal bacteria. Elimination of these organisms with antibiotics may lead to disappearance of the plasma cells and halting of the disease progression. Gilinsky et al. (1987)[61] make the point that a normal distal duodenal or jejunal biopsy virtually excludes IPSID. Once lymphoma has developed the outlook is poor. Treatment is by excisional surgery to remove or reduce the tumour bulk followed by radiotherapy and/or chemotherapy (Rambaud, 1983)[62].

## Burkitt-Like Lymphoma

The classical African Burkitt's lymphoma does not usually present in the gastrointestinal tract but a neoplasm which histologically closely resembles Burkitt's lymphoma commonly affects the terminal ileum in children in North Africa and the Middle East (Anaissie et al., 1985)[45]. These tumours have a strong association with Epstein–Barr virus. The neoplasms commonly present as large obstructing masses in the terminal ileum or as an intussusception.

The spread to mesenteric lymph nodes occurs early in the disease and is usually present at the time of presentation. Treatment is by debulking surgery followed by combination chemotherapy but the prognosis is poor (Rambaud, 1983)[62].

## Multiple Lymphomatous Polyposis (MLP)

MLP was first suggested by Cornes (1961)[63], and the largest series was published by Blackshaw (1980)[44]. In MLP the polyps can be found in the stomach, small or large intestine, frequently involving long ileocolic segments which may resemble a localised form of polyposis coli. Histologically the polyps consist of mucosal lymphoid nodules. The disease is associated with rapid deterioration and progression into the spleen and sometimes peripheral lymph nodes.

## Enteropathy-Associated T Cell Lymphoma

The association between malabsorption and intestinal lymphoma was recognised more than 50 years ago by Furley and McKee (1937)[64]. Gough et al. (1962)[65] established the association between coeliac disease and lymphoma and stated that lymphoma occurs as a complication rather than a cause of coeliac disease. Cooper et al. (1984)[66] review lymphoma in coeliac disease. They note an especially high risk in patients over 50 years of age in whom 10% develop lymphoma within 4 years of diagnosis. Isaacson et al. (1985)[47] demonstrated that these neoplasms are of T cell origin. Previously they had been described as malignant histiocytosis of the intestine but they are now called enteropathy-associated T cell lymphoma.

Grossly the neoplasms may occur as a single ulcerating mass or as multiple tumours in any part of the small intestine. The tumour may extend into the mesentery and large mesenteric nodes are common. Histologically the appearances are very variable and unlike other lymphomas they may be distorted by ulceration producing a mixed inflammatory infiltrate with only occasional foci of neoplastic cells. It is in these circumstances that the examination of other tissue from liver, spleen, bone marrow or mesenteric lymph nodes may help to establish the diagnosis. In some cases it is essential to examine large numbers of blocks in ulcerated areas to establish the diagnosis. Sometimes the cells appear as large immature blast cells with prominent nucleoli but in others the cells are pleomorphic and may have multiple nuclei. The adjacent mucosa will show features of villous atrophy, unless the patient is on a gluten-free diet. Cooper et al. (1980)[67] analysed the clinical presentation of lymphoma in coeliac disease which often presents as a deterioration of symptoms in a previously well-controlled coeliac patient. There is an average of about 8 years between diagnosis and malignant change. Some patients are not known to have coeliac disease before developing the tumour. This group may present insidiously or as an emergency with perforation or obstruction. Cooper et al. (1980)[67] suggest investigation by routine small bowel study but stress that diagnosis of lymphoma is often delayed and that 90% have very advanced disease at operation. They advise early operation if lymphoma is suspected.

Treatment is by surgical excision followed by combination chemotherapy and gluten-free diet.

## Smooth Muscle Tumours

It is difficult to assess accurately the frequency of smooth muscle intestinal tumours because they are often small and symptomless. The commonest site of symptomatic smooth muscle tumours is the small intestine where they may cause bleeding or obstruction or present with less clearly defined symptoms (Evans, 1985)[68]. It is important to realise that the distinction between benign and malignant tumours throughout the gastrointestinal tract is difficult on histological assessment. The size of the lesion together with the presence or absence of necrosis and mitotic activity are features which, in aggregate, may separate benign from malignant tumours (Morgan et al. 1990)[69].

Walsh and Mann (1984)[70] review smooth muscle tumours of the rectum and anal canal which may arise from the muscularis propria or from the muscularis mucosa. They may occur at any age and there is a slight predilection for males. Tumours which arise from the muscularis mucosa are benign, often asymptomatic and seldom measure more than 1 cm in diameter. There is no recurrence after local excision. Those arising from the muscularis propria may be either benign or malignant in behaviour and vary in size. They will commonly recur if treated by local excision and poorly differentiated leiomyosarcomas invariably develop distant metastases.

### Stromal Tumours

Malignant stromal tumours may be of muscle or neural origin but can be difficult to characterise. Ricci et al. (1987)[71] conclude that the majority of stromal sarcomas of the small intestine are of smooth muscle origin rather than of neural origin. De Schryver (1990)[72] tabulates the papers about immunohistochemical and electron microscopic features of epithelial and stromal tumours. He states that these markers are useful to separate epithelial from stromal tumours but are less useful in subdividing the stromal lesions. Kaposi's sarcoma (KS) used to be a very rare skin tumour in the UK and other Western countries but it is now seen much more frequently because it is the commonest tumour seen in patients with AIDS (Rotterdam and Sommers, 1985)[73]. It seems that the more marked the skin involvement with KS the more likely it is that there will be gastrointestinal involvement. KS involves the upper gastrointestinal tract more commonly than the lower (Kriegl and Friedman-Kien, 1988)[74]. Most patients with gastrointestinal KS are asymptomatic but it may cause bleeding, obstruction or perforation (Macho, 1988)[75]. The lesion is a malignant tumour of endothelial cell origin but requires a deep biopsy for diagnosis. Despite the apparent vascular nature of the lesion, bleeding after biopsy is very unusual (Mitsuyasu, 1988)[76].

## Vascular Abnormalities

True vascular neoplasms are rare and most intestinal vascular abnormalities take the form of haemangiomas or vascular malformations (Moore et al., 1976)[77]. Camilleri et al. (1984)[78] review vascular lesions which they classify into five groups: angiodysplasia (vascular ectasia), phlebectasia, telangiectasia, haemangioma and vascular connective tissue disorders (pseudoxanthoma elasticum and Ehlers–Danlos syndrome).

Boley and Brandt (1986)[79] give an excellent review of angiodysplasia. They point out that angiodysplasia is commonest in the right colon but it may occur elsewhere in the intestine and that it is usually associated with minor rather than major bleeding. They stress the relationship with cardiac disease, in particular aortic stenosis which is present in 25% of patients with angiodysplasia. Vase and Grove (1986)[80] describe the intestinal involvement in hereditary haemorrhagic telangiectasia.

Intestinal haemangioma is said to be the fifth most common benign small bowel "tumour" representing about 10% of cases (Miles et al., 1979)[81]. Colonic haemangiomas are rare and usually arise from the submucosal plexus but can show a variety of histological types (Lyon and Mantea, 1984)[82]. Diffuse cavernous haemangioma is a very rare variant and usually affects the pelvic colorectum and may extend to surrounding viscera (Taylor and Torrance, 1974)[83]. Lymphangiomas have been described in children and most usually affect the small rather than the large intestine. The tumours are often large but produce little in the way of symptoms (Whitehead, 1989)[84]. Lymphangiectasia is a more generalised disorder of the lymphatics of the mucous membrane and submucosa. This is a rare condition of young adults which leads to diarrhoea, weight loss and a protein-losing enteropathy. They have impaired cellular immunity probably due to loss of lymphocytes (Sorensen et al., 1985)[85].

## References

1. Olmsted WW, Ros PR, Hjermstad BM, McCarthy MJ, Dachman AH (1987) Tumors of the small intestine with little or no malignant pre-disposition. A review of the literature and report of 56 cases. Gastrointest Radiol 12:231–239
2. Spigelman AD, Murday V, Phillips RKS (1989) Cancer and the Peutz–Jeghers syndrome. Gut 30:1588–1590
3. Weiss NS, Yang CP (1987) Incidence of histologic types of cancer of the small intestine. JNCI 78:653–656
4. Taggart DP, Imrie CW (1987) A new pattern of histologic predominance and distribution of malignant diseases of the small intestine. Surg Gynecol Obstet 165:515–518
5. Johnson AM, Harman PK, Hanks JB (1985) Primary small bowel malignancies. Am Surg 51:31–36
6. Brophy C, Kahow CE (1989) Primary small bowel malignant tumors: unrecognised until emergency laparotomy. Am Surg 55:408–412
7. Maglinte DDT, Herlinger H (1989) Clinical radiology of the small intestine. Saunders, Philadelphia, pp 107–118
8. Tillotson CL, Geller SC, Kantrowitz L, Eckstein MR, Waltman AC, Athanasoulis CA

(1988) Small bowel hemorrhage: angiographic localisation and intervention. Gastrointest Radiol 13:207–211
9. Van Stolk R, Sivak MV, Petrini JL et al. (1987) Endoscopic management of upper gastrointestinal polyps and periampullary lesions in familial adenomatous polyposis and Gardner's syndrome. Endoscopy 19:19–22
10. Lewis BS, Waye JD (1988) Chronic gastrointestinal bleeding of obscure origin: role of small bowel enteroscopy. Gastroenterology 94:1117–1120
11. Bentley E, Chandrasona P, Radia R, Cohn H (1989) Generalised juvenile polyposis with carcinoma. Am J Gastroenterol 84:1456–1459
12. Richards ME, Rickert RR, Nance FC (1989) Crohn's disease-associated carcinoma: a poorly recognised complication of inflammatory bowel disease. Am Surg 209:764–773
13. Fishman MJ, Jeejeeboy KN, Gopinath N, Girotti MJ, Yeung EY, Cullen JR (1990) Small intestinal villous adenocarcinoma and coeliac disease. Am J Gastroenterol 85:748–751
14. Walter JB, Israel MS (1979) Disturbances of endocrine function. In: General pathology, 5th edn. J.B. Walter and M.S. Israel (eds). Churchill Livingstone, Edinburgh, p 452
15. William ED, Sandler M (1963) The classification of tumours. Lancet i:238–239
16. Moertel SG, Sauer WG, Dockerty MB (1961) Life history of carcinoid tumour of the small intestine. Cancer 14:908–912
17. Willander E, Portellagomez G, Grimelius L, Westermark P (1977) Argentaffin and argyrophil reaction of human gastrointestinal carcinoids. Gastroenterology 73:733–736
18. Marks C (1979) Carcinoid tumour. A clinico-pathologic study. G.K. Hall, Boston
19. Sanders RJ (1973) In: Carcinoids of the gastrointestinal tract. C.C. Thomas. Springfield, Illinois, pp 1–110
20. Morgan JG, Marks C, Hearn D (1974) Carcinoid tumours of the gastrointestinal tract. Ann Surg 180:720–727
21. Creutzfeldt W, Stöckmann F (1987) Carcinoids and carcinoid syndrome. Am J Med 32:4–15
22. Norheim I, Öberg K, Theodorsson-Norheim E et al. (1987) Malignant carcinoid tumors: an analysis of 103 patients with regard to tumor localization, hormone production and survival. Ann Surg 206:115–125
23. Grahame-Smith DG (1987) What is the cause of the carcinoid flush? Gut 28:1413–1416
24. Woods HF, Bax NDS, Smith JAR (1985) Small bowel carcinoid tumors. World J Surg 9:921–929
25. Bukowski RM, Johnson KG, Peterson RF et al. (1987) A phase II trial of combination with chemotherapy in patients with metastatic carcinoid tumors: a southwest oncology group study. Cancer 60:2891–2895
26. Souquet JC, Sassolas G, Forichon J, Champetier P, Partensky C, Chayvialle JA (1987) Clinical and hormonal effects of a long-acting somatostatin analogue in pancreatic endocrine tumors and in carcinoid syndrome. Cancer 59:1654–1660
27. Zollinger RM, Ellison EM (1955) Primary peptic ulceration of the jejunum associated with islet cell tumours of the pancreas. Ann Surg 142:704–728
28. Walsh JH, Grossman MI (1975) Gastrin. N Engl J Med 291:1324–1332, 1377–1384
29. Oberhelman HA (1972) Excisional therapy for ulcerogenic tumors of the duodenum: long-term results. Arch Surg 104:447–453
30. Soergel KW (1975) Hormonally mediated diarrhoea. N Engl J Med 292:970–972
31. Gander OP, Weir GC, Sollinder JS et al. (1977) Somastatinoma – a somastatin-containing tumor of the endocrine pancreas. N Engl J Med 296:963–967
32. Marcus FS, Friedman MA, Callen PW, Churg A, Harbour J (1980) Successful therapy of an ACTH-producing gastric carcinoid APUD tumor. Report of a case and review of the literature. Cancer 46:1263–1269
33. Herata Y, Sakomotu N, Yiamotu H, Matsukna S, Imora H, Okada S (1976) Gastric carcinoid with ectopic production of ACTH and beta MSH. Cancer 37:377–385
34. Welbourn RB (1977) Current status of apudomas. Ann Surg 185:1–12
35. Freeman C, Berg JW, Cutler SJ (1972) Occurrence and progress of extranodal lymphomas. Cancer 29:252–260
36. Wright DH, Isaacson PG (1983) Biopsy pathology of the lymphoreticular system. Chapman and Hall, London
37. Lewin KJ, Ranchod M, Dorfman RF (1978) Lymphomas of the gastrointestinal tract. Cancer 42:693–707
38. Cornes JS (1967) Hodgkin's disease of the gastrointestinal tract. Proc R Soc Med 60:732–733

39. Wright DH, Isaacson PG (1989) Gut-associated lymphoid tumours. In: Gastrointestinal and oesophageal biopsy. R. Whitehead (ed). Churchill Livingstone, Edinburgh, pp 644–661
40. Hall PA, Jass JR, Levison DA, Morson BC, Shepherd NA, Sobin L, Stansfield AG (1988) Classifying primary gut lymphomas. Lancet ii:1317
41. Aozasa K, Ueda T, Kurata A et al. (1988) Prognostic value of histologic and clinical factors in 56 patients with gastrointestinal lymphomas. Cancer 61:309–315
42. Khojasteh A, Haghsenass M, Haghighi P (1983) Immuno-proliferative small intestinal disease. A Third World lesion. N Engl J Med 308:1401–1405
43. Matuchansky C, Touchard G, Babin P, Lemaire M, Cogne M, Preud-Homme JL (1988) Diffuse small intestinal lymphoid infiltration in non-immunodeficient adults from Western Europe. Gastroenterology 95:470–477
44. Blackshaw AJ (1980) Non-Hodgkin's lymphoma of the gut. In: Recent advances in gastrointestinal pathology 13. R. Wright (ed). Saunders, Eastbourne
45. Anaissie E, Geha S, Allam C, Jabbour J, Khaky KM, Salem P (1985) Burkitt's lymphoma in the Middle East. A study of 34 cases. Cancer 56:2539–2543
46. Kanavaros P, Lavergne A, Galian A et al. (1988) A primary immunoblastic T malignant lymphoma of the small bowel, with azurophilic intracytoplasmic granules. Am J Surg Pathol 12:641–647
47. Isaacson PG, O'Connor NTJ, Spencer J et al. (1985) Malignant histocytosis of the intestine. A T cell lymphoma. Lancet ii:688–691
48. Al-Bahrani ZR, Al-Mondhiri H, Bakir F, Al-Saleem T (1983) Clinical and pathologic subtypes of primary intestinal lymphoma: experience with 132 patients over a 14-year period. Cancer 52:1666–1672
49. Green JA, Dawson AA, Jones PF, Blunt PW (1979) The presentation of gastrointestinal lymphomas: study of a population. Br J Surg 66:798–801
50. Baildam AD, Williams GT, Schofield PF (1989) Abdominal lymphoma. J R Soc Med 82:657–660
51. Seigel MJ, Evans SJ, Balfe DM (1988) Small bowel disease in children: diagnosis with CT. Pediatr Radiol 169:127–130
52. Grody WW, Weiss LM, Warnike RA, Magidson JG, Hu E, Lewin KJ (1985) Gastrointestinal lymphomas: immunohistochemical studies on the cell of origin. Am J Surg Pathol 9:328–337
53. Hockey MS, Powell J, Crocker J, Fielding JWL (1987) Primary gastric lymphoma. Br J Surg 74:483–487
54. Perrin T, Blackledge G (1986) Gastrointestinal lymphomas. In: Gastrointestinal oncology. J.W.L. Fielding, J.J.Priestman (eds). Castle House, Tunbridge Wells, pp 237–255
55. Zwigler JL (1984) Non-Hodgkin's lymphoma in 90 homosexual men: relationship to generalised lymphadenopathy and acquired immunodeficiency syndrome. N Engl J Med 311:565–571
56. Joachim HL, Cooper ML, Hellman GC (1985) Lymphoma in men at high risk for acquired immune deficiency syndrome. Cancer 56:2831–2842
57. Kaplan LD, Wofsy CB, Volberding PA (1987) Treatment of patients with acquired immunodeficiency syndrome and associated manifestations. JAMA 257:1367–1374
58. Hoover R, Fraumeni FR (1973) Risk of cancer in renal-transplant recipients. Lancet ii:55–57
59. Galian A, Leicester MJ, Scott J, Bogwell C, Mutuchansky C, Rambod JC (1977) Pathological study of alpha chain disease with a special emphasis on evolution. Cancer 39:2081–2101
60. Smith WJ, Price SK, Isaacson PG (1987) Immunoglobulin gene rearrangement in immunoproliferative small intestinal disease (IPSID). J Clin Pathol 40:1291–1297
61. Gilinsky NH, Novis VH, Wright JP, Dent DM, King H, Marks IN (1987) Immunoproliferative small-intestinal disease: clinical features and outcome in 30 cases. Medicine 66:438–446
62. Rambaud JC (1983) Small intestinal lymphomas and alpha chain disease. Clin Gastroenterol 12:743–766
63. Cornes JS (1961) Multiple lymphomatous polyposis of the gastrointestinal tract. Cancer 14:249–257
64. Furley NH, McKee FP (1937) The clinical and biochemical syndrome of lymphadenoma and coeliac disease involving the mesenteric lymph glands. Br Med J i:3972–3980
65. Gough KR, Reid AE, Nyesh AR (1962) Intestinal reticulosis as a complication of idiopathic steatorrhoea. Gut 3:232–239

66. Cooper BT, Holmes GKT, Cooke WT (1984) Cancer in celiac disease. Surv Dig Dis 2:52–59
67. Cooper BT, Holmes GKT, Ferguson R, Cooke WT (1980) Celiac disease and malignancy. Medicine 59:249–261
68. Evans HL (1985) Smooth muscle tumours of the gastrointestinal tract. A study of 56 cases for a minimum of 10 years. Cancer 56:2242–2250
69. Morgan BK, Compton C, Talbeart M, Gallagher WJ, Wood WC (1990) Benign smooth muscle tumours of the gastrointestinal tract: a 24-year experience. Ann Surg 211:63–66
70. Walsh TH, Mann CV (1984) Smooth muscle neoplasms of the rectum and anal canal. Br J Surg 71:597–599
71. Ricci A, Ciccarelli O, Cartun RW, Newcomb P (1987) A clinicopathologic and immunohistochemical study of 16 patients with small intestine leiomyosarcoma: limited utility of immunophenotyping. Cancer 60:1790–1799
72. De Schryver K (1990) Small intestine pathology. Curr Opin Gastroenterol 6:258–263
73. Rotterdam HZ, Sommers SC (1985) Alimentary tract biopsy lesions in the acquired immunodeficiency syndrome. Pathology 17:181–192
74. Kriegl RL, Friedman-Kien AE (1988) Kaposi's sarcoma in AIDS. Diagnosis and treatment. In: AIDS: etiology, diagnosis, treatment and prevention, 2nd edn. V.T. DeVita, S. Hellman, S.A. Rosenberg (eds). Lippincott, New York, pp 245–261
75. Macho JR (1988) Gastrointestinal surgery in the AIDS patient. Gastroenterol Clin North Am 17:563–571
76. Mitsuyashu RT (1988) Kaposi's sarcoma in the acquired immunodeficiency syndrome. Infect Dis Clin North Am 2:511–523
77. Moore JD, Thompson NN, Appleman HD, Foley D (1976) Arterio-venous malformations of the gastrointestinal tract. Arch Surg 111:381–389
78. Camilleri M, Chadwick VS, Hodgson HJF (1984) Vascular anomalies of the gastrointestinal tract. Hepatogastroenterology 31:149–153
79. Boley SJ, Brandt LJ (1986) Vascular ectasias of the colon. Dig Dis Sci 31:26S–42S
80. Vase P, Grove O (1986) Gastrointestinal lesions in hereditary hemorrhagic telangiectasia. Gastroenterology 91:1079–1083
81. Miles RM, Crawford D, Duras S (1979) The small bowel tumour problem. An assessment based on a 20-year experience with 116 cases. Ann Surg 185:732–738
82. Lyon DT, Mantea AG (1984) Large bowel haemangioma. Dis Colon Rectum 27:404–414
83. Taylor TV, Torrance HB (1974) Haemangiomatosis of the gastrointestinal tract. Br J Surg 61:236–238
84. Whitehead R (1989) Gastrointestinal and oesophageal biopsy. Churchill Livingstone, Edinburgh,
85. Sorensen RU, Halpin TC, Abramowsky CR et al. (1985) Intestinal lymphangiectasia and thymic hypoplasia. Clin Exp Immunol 59:217–226

# 11 Benign Epithelial Tumours and Polyps

Morson and Dawson (1990)[1] define an intestinal polyp as a mucosal projection into the lumen of the bowel. This does not indicate the underlying nature of the lesion. The polyps can be single or multiple and if multiple they may be in small numbers or in hundreds or thousands – polyposis. Different types of polyp are produced by different pathological processes: neoplasia leads to adenoma, inflammation to an inflammatory polyp, malformation leads to juvenile and Peutz–Jeghers polyps and dysmaturation to the hyperplastic (metaplastic) polyp. The gross and microscopic features of these different types are beautifully illustrated in Morson's colour atlas (1988)[2].

## Adenoma

Adenoma is a benign neoplasm of glandular epithelium which may be defined as a circumscribed focus of dysplastic epithelium (Konishi and Morson, 1982)[3]. Tiny adenomas are sessile and large adenomas may be sessile or pedunculated. The pedicle contains submucosa and sizeable vessels. The transition from adjacent normal mucosa is abrupt. Autopsy surveys indicate that adenomas are evenly distributed throughout the colon and rectum (Williams et al., 1982)[4]. One study has shown that adenomas are frequent at the extremes of the large bowel (Vatn and Stalsberg, 1982)[5]. In younger subjects, the left colon and rectum are more often populated by adenomas whilst with increasing years the right colon becomes the site of predilection (Gerharz et al., 1987)[6]. It is interesting to see that whilst adenomas are uncommon before the age of 30 their frequency increases significantly later in life but they plateau beyond the seventh decade (Bernstein et al., 1985)[7]. Although there are some anomalies, the prevalence of adenomas in a country correlates with the incidence of colorectal carcinoma (Correa, 1978)[8].

Adenomas are more common in males in all regions of the large bowel whereas the sex ratio for cancer excluding the rectum is almost 1 : 1. This may indicate that females are less likely to produce adenomas but once formed they are more likely to progress to malignancy. Morson and Bussey (1985)[9] showed that individuals presenting with one or more adenomas are at increased risk of producing additional adenomas. By 15 years from the initial presentation the cumulative risk of further adenomas is 50%. Adenomas occur with increased frequency in patients belonging to colorectal cancer families (Lovatt, 1976)[10]. Hill et al. (1977)[11] postulated that both genetic and environmental factors are responsible for the development of adenoma and its subsequent progression to carcinoma. Burt et al. (1985)[12] present evidence that leaves little doubt that genetic influences are the principal factors leading to adenoma formation.

The World Health Organization (WHO) international histological classification (Morson and Sobin, 1976)[13] recognises three types of adenoma; tubular, villous and tubulovillous. Muto et al. (1975)[14] showed that adenomas may undergo malignant change. Wolff and Shinya (1975)[15] show that sessile lesions are more likely to be malignant than polypoid lesions. Muto et al. (1985)[16] draw our attention to the flat adenoma which may be difficult to diagnose colonoscopically. They review 33 small flat lesions less than 1 cm and 14 of these showed severe dysplasia. They postulate that these may be important in the adenoma–carcinoma sequence. A review by Day (1984)[17] states that the likelihood of malignancy developing in an adenoma increases with villous pattern, size and severity of dysplasia. Grinnell and Lane (1985)[18] record invasive malignant change in 32% of villous tumours compared to 3% in tubular adenomas. They found malignant features in less than 1% of tumours less than 1 cm in size but 14% in tumours greater than 2.5 cm and a similar finding comes from Muto et al. (1975)[14]. Morson and Sobin (1976)[13] lay down grading of adenomas into mild, moderate and severe dysplasia and give criteria. Despite this, there is no doubt that grading is subjective with only modest interobserver agreement (Brown et al., 1985)[19]. Goh and Jass (1986)[20] showed that severity of dysplasia in an adenoma correlated with DNA aneuploidy on flow cytometry.

WHO nomenclature has standardised a confused terminology regarding dysplasia in adenoma and early carcinoma. Early carcinoma should only be used if there is extension through the lamina propria. Morson and Dawson (1990)[1] reject the terms carcinoma-in-situ, intramucosal carcinoma and focal carcinoma and state that these changes should be termed adenoma with severe dysplasia. This assumes great significance because of the development of colonoscopic polypectomy. All tumours localised to the mucosa with no evidence of invasion can be treated satisfactorily by colonoscopic polypectomy because they do not metastasise (Morson et al., 1977)[21]. On the other hand, Cooper (1983)[22] shows that 10% of true early carcinomas, i.e. with invasion, have lymph node involvement. Muto et al. (1987)[23] found that this increased to 30% if there was evidence of lymphatic invasion in the polyp. There is a low risk of lymph node metastases and local recurrence after polypectomy if the stalk is involved down to the level of section (Cooper, 1983)[22]. Total excision of the entire polyp is the correct treatment and allows an adequate histological examination. There is no place for endoscopic biopsy of excisable colonic polyps. Sawada et al. (1989)[24] recommend a standard bowel resection if the polyp is poorly differentiated or shows lymphatic invasion but believe that stalk invasion down to the section margin does not require further operation if the colonoscopist believes the resection is total.

Bussey (1975)[25] gives an excellent overview of the familial adenomatous polyposis syndromes. They are discussed further in Chapter 12.

## Peutz–Jeghers Polyposis

Peutz–Jeghers syndrome is a rare autosomal dominant disease characterised by hamartomatous polyps in the gastrointestinal tract and by mucocutaneous melanin pigmentation (Peutz, 1921; Jeghers, 1944)[26,27]. The polyps are found most frequently in the small bowel but may occur in the stomach and colon concurrently. In the usual type there are multiple polyps throughout the gastrointestinal tract. Bartholomew et al. (1957)[28] describe the basic hamartomatous abnormality involving the muscularis mucosa which appears as tree-like branching bundles of smooth muscle covered by mucosa of the type native to that part of the bowel from which the polyp has arisen. There is an association with carcinoma outside the gastrointestinal tract especially in breast, ovary and cervix (Giardiello et al., 1987)[29]. There is a well-recognised predisposition to intestinal cancer (Dozois et al., 1969)[30].

Shepherd et al. (1987)[31] highlighted epithelial misplacement commonly seen in these polyps which can be mistaken for malignant invasion and suggested that the cancer risk may have been exaggerated in the past. Spigelman et al. (1989)[32] assessed 72 patients retrospectively and confirmed that there was an excess of both intestinal and extraintestinal carcinomas. They suggest that there is evidence of hamartoma–carcinoma sequence in Peutz–Jeghers syndrome. The life expectancy of sufferers is shortened by the high incidence of cancer.

## Juvenile Polyps

Horrilleno et al. (1957)[33] pointed out that a juvenile polyp was a specific pathological entity and that it is the commonest type of polyp in children. Knox et al. (1960)[34] stated that 80% occurred in children under 10 years of age. The polyps are multiple in about 30% of patients. McColl et al. (1964)[35] suggested there was a familial tendency in juvenile polyps. Bussey (1970)[36] reported that other congenital abnormalities may be associated occasionally.

Juvenile polyps are non-neoplastic epithelial polyps with a narrow stalk and a red spherical head. They are composed of tissue indigenous to the site of origin but arranged in a haphazard manner. The histological appearance is typical with irregular cystic glands separated by abundant lamina propria covered with smooth surface epithelium (Knox et al., 1960)[34]. They are probably examples of hamartomata (Morson, 1988)[2]. Bartnik et al. (1986)[37] treated 48 children with juvenile polyps by colonoscopic removal, without recurrence. They do not believe that single polyps require follow-up colonoscopy.

The usual presenting symptom is rectal bleeding. Perisic (1987)[38] found 45 polyps by colonoscopy in 71 children investigated for bleeding; 83% of these were of juvenile type. In juvenile polyposis there is an increased risk of malignancy but the magnitude of the risk is probably low (Jarvinen and Franssila, 1984)[39]. The cancers appear between the ages of 20 and 40 years.

## Hyperplastic (Metaplastic) Polyps

Morson (1962)[40] differentiated metaplastic polyps from adenoma because of the clear histological differences. Hyperplastic or metaplastic polyps are better termed dysmaturation polyps because the underlying defect involves elongation of the proliferative component of the crypt. The migration of maturing cells from the proliferative component is slowed and the crypt columnar cells show premature or inappropriate cytoplasmic maturation (Morson, 1962)[40]. The surface epithelium is serrated or saw-toothed. They show a striking predilection for the rectum and the left colon (Correa, 1978)[8]. They are typically small, rarely more than 0.5 cm but large hyperplastic polyps have been described in young people (Williams et al., 1980)[41]. They are more common in high risk areas for colorectal cancer (Stemmermann and Yatani, 1973)[42]. This observation suggests that hyperplastic polyps are caused by an environmental factor which is concentrated in the left colon, particularly with a high risk population for colorectal cancer. Eide (1986)[43] has shown that they are 17 times more common in segments of large bowel containing cancer compared with autopsy-derived segments matched for site, age and sex. They are more common and more likely to be multiple in patients with colorectal adenomas. There is a low incidence of dysplasia observed in hyperplastic polyps and rarely frank carcinomas can be seen (Cooper et al., 1979)[44]. Some authorities suggest that the risk of cancer in patients with multiple hyperplastic polyps may be higher than the risk in the general population (Bengoachea et al., 1987)[45]. Waye (1988)[46] doubts that hyperplastic polyps are markers of high risk.

## Inflammatory Polyps

These are non-neoplastic proliferations of either mucosa or granulation tissue which may be due to various injuries of the colorectal epithelium (Dukes, 1954)[47]. They are seen in ulcerative colitis, Crohn's disease, schistosomiasis and ischaemic bowel. Edling and Eklöf (1961)[48] convincingly rejected the hypothesis that inflammatory polyposis in ulcerative colitis predisposed to malignancy. Kelly et al. (1986)[49] give a review of inflammatory polyps in ulcerative colitis and confirm that they are unrelated to malignant transformation but ulcerate and tend to be associated with bleeding.

In children, benign lymphoid hyperplasia with small colonic nodules produces a type of polyposis (Morson and Dawson, 1990)[1]. It is usually considered to be asymptomatic but Kaplan et al. (1984)[50] suggested that it was a cause of lower gastrointestinal bleeding.

# References


1. Morson BC, Dawson IMP (1990) Gastrointestinal pathology, 3rd edn. Blackwell Scientific, Oxford
2. Morson BC (1988) Colour atlas of gastrointestinal pathology. Oxford University Press, Oxford
3. Konishi F, Morson BC (1982) Pathology of colorectal adenomas. J Clin Pathol 35:830–841
4. Williams AR, Balasooriya BAW, Day DW (1982) Polyps and cancer of the large intestine. Necropsy study in Liverpool. Gut 23:835–842
5. Vatn MH, Stalsberg H (1982) The prevalence of polyps of the large intestine in Oslo: an autopsy study. Cancer 49:819–825
6. Gerhartz CD, Gabbert H, Krummel F (1987) Age-dependent shift to the right in the localisation of colorectal adenomas. Virchows Arch [A] 411:591–598.
7. Bernstein MA, Feczko PJ, Halpert RD, Simms SM, Ackerman LV (1985) Distribution of colonic polyps. Increased incidence of proximal lesions in older patient. Radiology 155:35–38
8. Correa P (1978) Epidemiology of polyps and cancer. In: The pathogenesis of colorectal cancer. B.C. Morson (ed). Saunders, Philadelphia, pp 126–152
9. Morson BC, Bussey HJR (1985) Magnitude of risk for cancer in patients with colorectal adenomas. Br J Surg 72:523–528
10. Lovatt E (1976) Family studies in cancer of the colon and rectum. Br J Surg 63:13–18
11. Hill MJ, Morson BC, Bussey HJR (1977) Aetiology of adenoma–carcinoma sequence in large bowel. Lancet i:535–538
12. Burt RW, Bishop DT, Cannon LA, Dowdle MA, Lee RG, Skolnick MH (1985) Dominant inheritance of adenomatous colonic polyps and colorectal cancer. N Engl J Med 312:1540–1544
13. Morson BC, Sobin LH (1976) International histological classification of tumours, No. 15. Histological typing of intestinal tumours. World Health Organization, Geneva
14. Muto T, Bussey HJR, Morson BC (1975) The evolution of cancer of the colon and rectum. Cancer 36:2251–2263
15. Wolff WI, Shinya H (1975) Definitive treatment of "malignant" polyps of the colon. Ann Surg 182:516–525
16. Muto T, Kamiya J, Sawada T et al. (1985) Small "flat adenoma" of the large bowel with special reference to its clinicopathologic features Dis Colon Rectum 28:847–851
17. Day DW (1984) The adenoma–carcinoma sequence. Scand J Gastroenterol 19 (Suppl 104):99–108
18. Grinnell RS, Lane N (1958) Benign and malignant adenomatous polyps and papillary adenomas of the colon and rectum. An analysis of 1856 tumours in 1335 patients. Surg Gynecol Obstet 106:519–538
19. Brown LJR, Smeeton NC, Dixon MF (1985) Assessment of dysplasia in colorectal adenomas: an observer variation and morphometric study. J Clin Pathol 38:174–179
20. Goh HS, Jass JR (1986) DNA content and the adenoma–carcinoma sequence in the colorectum. J Clin Pathol 39:387–392
21. Morson BC, Bussey HJR, Samoorian S (1977) Policy of local excision for early cancer of the colon and rectum. Gut 18:1045–1050
22. Cooper HS (1983) Surgical pathology of endoscopically removed malignant polyps of the colon and rectum. Am J Surg Pathol 7:613–623
23. Muto T, Konishi F, Sawada T et al. (1987) Colonoscopic polypectomy as a tool for management of colonic polyps and detection of new lesions. Ann Acad Med Singapore 16:427–431
24. Sawada T, Hojo K, Moriya Y (1989) Colonoscopic management of focal and early colorectal carcinoma. Baillière Clin Gastroenterol Colorectal Cancer 3:627–645
25. Bussey HJR (1975) Familial polyposis coli. Johns Hopkins University Press, Baltimore.
26. Peutz JLA (1921) On a very remarkable case of familial polyposis of the mucous membrane of the intestinal tract and nasopharynx accompanied by peculiar pigmentations of the skin and mucous membrane. Ned Tijdschr Geneeskd 10:134–146
27. Jeghers H (1944) Pigmentation of the skin. N Engl J Med 231:88

28. Bartholomew LG, Dahlin D, Waugh JM (1957) Intestinal polyposis associated with mucocutaneous melanin pigmentation (Peutz–Jeghers syndrome). Gastroenterology 32:434–451
29. Giardiello FM, Welsh SB, Hamilton SR et al. (1987) Increased risk of cancer in Peutz–Jeghers syndrome. N Engl J Med 316:1511–1514
30. Dozois RR, Judd ES, Dahlin DC, Bartholomew LG (1969) The Peutz–Jeghers syndrome: is there a predisposition to the development of intestinal malignancy? Arch Surg 98:509–516
31. Shepherd NA, Bussey HJR, Jass JR (1987) Epithelial misplacement in Peutz–Jeghers polyps: a diagnostic pitfall. Am J Surg Pathol 11:743–749
32. Spigelman AD, Murday V, Phillips RKS (1989) Cancer and the Peutz–Jeghers syndrome. Gut 30:1588–1590
33. Horrilleno EG, Eckert C, Ackerman LV (1957) Polyps of the rectum and colon in children. Cancer 10:1210–1220
34. Knox WG, Miller RE, Begg CF, Zintel HA (1960) Juvenile polyps of the colon: a clinicopathologic analysis of 75 polyps in 43 patients. Surgery 48:201–210
35. McColl I, Bussey HJR, Veale AM, Morson BC (1964) Juvenile polyposis coli. Proc R Soc Med 57:896–897
36. Bussey HJR (1970) Gastrointestinal polyposis. Gut 11:970–978
37. Bartnik W, Botruk E, Ryzko J, Rondio H, Rasinski A, Orlowska J (1986) Short- and long-term results of colonic polypectomy in children. Gastrointest Endosc 32:389–392
38. Perisic VN (1987) Colorectal polyps: an important cause of rectal bleeding. Arch Dis Child 62:188–203
39. Jarvinen H, Franssila KO (1984) Familial juvenile polyposis coli: increased risk of colorectal cancer. Gut 25:792–800
40. Morson BC (1962) Some peculiarities in the histology of intestinal polyps. Dis Colon Rectum 5:337–344
41. Williams GT, Arthur JF, Bussey HJR, Morson BC (1980) Metaplastic polyps and polyposis of the colorectum. Histopathology 4:115–170
42. Stemmermann GN, Yatani R (1973) Diverticulosis and polyps of the large intestine. A necropsy study of Hawaii Japanese. Cancer 31:1260–1270
43. Eide TJ (1986) Prevalence and morphological features of adenomas of the large intestine in individuals with and without colorectal carcinoma. Histopathology 10:111–118
44. Cooper HS, Patchchefsky AS, Marks G (1979) Adenomatous and carcinomatous changes within hyperplastic colonic epithelium. Dis Colon Rectum 22:152–156
45. Bengoachea O, Martinez-Penuela TM, Larrinaju B, Valendi J, Borda F (1987) Hyperplastic polyposis of the colorectum and adenocarcinoma in a 24-year-old man. Am J Surg Pathol 11:323–327
46. Waye JD (1988) Hyperplastic colon polyps – are they markers? Ann Intern Med 109:851–852
47. Dukes CE (1954) The surgical pathology of ulcerative colitis. Ann R Coll Surg Engl 14:389–400
48. Edling NP, Eklöf O (1961) Radiological findings and prognosis in ulcerative colitis. Acta Chir Scand 121:299–308
49. Kelly JK, Langevin JM, Price LM, Marshfield VB, Share S, Blustein P (1986) Giant and symptomatic inflammatory polyps of the colon in idiopathic inflammatory bowel disease. Am J Surg Pathol 10:420–428
50. Kaplan B, Benson J, Rothstein F, Dahms B, Halpin T (1984) Lymphonodular hyperplasia of the colon as a pathologic finding in children with lower gastrointestinal bleeding. J Pediatr Gastroenterol Nutr 3:704–708

# 12 Large Bowel Carcinoma

## Epidemiology and Pathogenesis

The incidence of large bowel carcinoma varies greatly between countries but it is common in most developed countries (Boyle et al., 1985)[1]. In the UK it stands second in frequency as a cause of death amongst malignant diseases (Office of Population Censuses and Surveys, 1986)[2]. Levin and Dozois (1991)[3] report a similar prevalence in the United States. They note a change in anatomical distribution of large bowel cancer in the last 40 years with an increase in right colonic tumours and a decrease in rectal tumours. At present about 60% of the tumours are in the rectum or sigmoid colon.

It has been suggested that the difference in geographical prevalence may be related to diet (Wynder and Shigematsu, 1967)[4]. Burkitt (1975)[5] suggested that a high incidence of large bowel carcinoma was associated with a lack of dietary fibre. Others have suggested that a high intake of animal fat and meat is causative (Nigro et al., 1975)[6]. It is postulated that the dietary fat alters the bile acids and colonic bacteria so as to induce changes towards intraluminal carcinogens (Hill, 1975)[7]. These issues are reviewed by Wargovich et al. (1988)[8].

Muto et al. (1975)[9] review the situation with regard to the development of large bowel cancer and suggest that most carcinomas develop from pre-existing adenomas, the so-called adenoma–carcinoma sequence. The evidence suggesting that most carcinomas arise from pre-existing adenomas is strong but circumstantial. Some of this evidence is as follows:

1. The presence of adenomas in resection specimens of colorectal cancer is six times as common as in similar specimens resected for non-malignant disease (Eide, 1986)[10].
2. The risk of a metachronous carcinoma is doubled in patients if the original resection specimen contained adenomas in addition to the carcinoma (Bussey et al., 1967)[11].
3. In patients with synchronous carcinoma, additional adenomas are found in 75% of specimens (Heald and Lockhart–Mummery, 1972)[12].
4. In some adenomas it is possible to see foci of malignant change and in some carcinomas there is evidence of a pre-existing adenoma (Ekelund and Lindström, 1974)[13].
5. Adenomas occur at an earlier age than carcinoma by approximately 5–10 years (Correa, 1978)[14].

6. Adenomas are larger and more numerous in patients from those geographical areas where there is a high incidence of large bowel carcinoma (Clark et al., 1985)[15].
7. There is an increase in dysplasia in aneuploid adenomas (Goh and Jass, 1986)[16]
8. Removal of adenomas reduces the incidence of cancer in the cleared segment of large bowel (Gilbertsen and Nelms, 1978)[17].

Large bowel cancer is usually a disease of the older patient but there are some families in whom there is a genetic predisposition. These patients are younger with a greater tendency to right colonic and multiple lesions. The non-polyposis cancer family syndromes are reviewed by Lynch et al. (1988)[18].

Premalignant conditions include ulcerative colitis, Crohn's disease and familial adenomatous polyposis (FAP). Malignant transformation in ulcerative colitis only occurs after many years and is much more likely when the colitis is extensive (Hordijk and Shivananda, 1989)[19]. Sugita et al. (1991)[20] assess the average interval between the onset of colitis and malignant transformation as being 21 years. Regular colonoscopy has been accepted as a screening method to detect cancer in longstanding ulcerative colitis but this concept is now seriously challenged. The evidence is reviewed by Gyde (1991)[21]. Greenstein et al. (1981)[22] believe that the cancer risk is similar in ulcerative colitis and Crohn's disease.

Familial adenomatous polyposis (FAP) is inherited as a Mendelian dominant and is a cause of about 1% of colorectal cancers (Mecklin, 1987)[23]. Variations from the classical syndrome exist. Gardner (1951)[24] recorded epidermoid cysts, exostoses and fibrous tumours as associates and later noted dental abnormalities (Gardner, 1962)[25]. Smith (1958)[26] reported desmoid tumours, usually in the anterior abdominal wall, as an association and suggested the term "Gardner's syndrome" for FAP associated with mesodermal abnormalities. The association between FAP and neural tumours has been termed Turcot's syndrome. These patients have café au lait pigmentation of the skin in addition (Turcot, 1959)[27]. Alm and Licznerski (1973)[28] have presented evidence to show that there is no genetic distinction between patients with extracolonic manifestations and those without such lesions in FAP. Van Stolk et al. (1987)[29] confirmed that duodenal adenomas were common in FAP and predominantly affected the periampullary region. Malignant transformation of one of the colonic adenomas would be inevitable, but many patients are diagnosed and treated by the appropriate surgery before malignant change occurs. The extracolonic manifestations of duodenal adenoma, desmoid tumours and fibromatosis have become the commonest cause of death (Jagelman et al., 1988)[30]. A further association of diagnostic use is the discovery of pigmented patches in the retina (CHRPE) (Diaz-Lopez and Menezo, 1987)[31]. A book reviewing the present state of knowledge in all aspects of FAP gives a good overview of the many facets of this condition (Herrera, 1989)[32].

Genetic abnormalities have been discovered in relationship to carcinoma of the colon. Deletion in the short arm of chromosome 5 was first noted in relationship to polyposis (Bodmer et al., 1987)[33]. In sporadic carcinomas there are multiple chromosomal abnormalities including chromosome 5q deletion as an early event (Vogelstein et al., 1988)[34]. Fearon and

Vogelstein (1990)[35] summarised the present knowledge which indicates a multiple genetic abnormality pathway in colorectal carcinogenesis including deletions on chromosome 17 and 18 as well as K-*ras* oncogene amplification. Fearon et al. (1990)[36] identified a short area on chromosome 18q which is absent in most tumours and have called it DCC (deleted in colon cancer).

The prognosis of large bowel cancer has only improved slightly this century but both an operating surgeon and a pathologist can give guidance as to prognosis in the individual patient (Schofield et al., 1986)[37].

Large bowel tumours may be multiple. The rate of synchronous malignant tumours varies in different reports from 3% to 12% (Cunliffe et al., 1984)[38]. For this reason, it is now generally agreed that total colonoscopy, either before surgery or shortly after operation, is indicated in all patients with large bowel tumour (Isler et al., 1987)[39].

## Pathology

Early in the twentieth century, Miles (1910)[40] showed in detail the potential lymphatic spread in relationship to rectal cancer. Dukes (1930)[41] showed that the more important mode of lymphatic spread was along the inferior mesenteric vessels and from this evolved a pathological classification which had prognostic significance (Dukes, 1940)[42]. This was an ABC classification in which A was an invasive tumour confined to the wall of the rectum, B was a tumour spreading outside the rectal serosa and C was a tumour with lymph gland metastases. Dukes (1945)[43] proposed the same system for colonic tumours.

Other ABC systems were proposed by Kirklin et al. (1949)[44] and Astler and Coller (1954)[45] but unfortunately this caused confusion because the stages were dissimilar to those proposed by Dukes. Turnbull et al. (1967)[46], recognising that this system of classification made no allowance for other areas of spread, proposed a clinicopathological classification retaining Dukes' A, B and C but adding category D when there was evidence of distant spread or extensive local spread. It is now well established that many cases have liver metastases at presentation (Cedermark et al., 1977)[47]. Bacon and Jackson (1953)[48] showed that 5% of patients had pulmonary metastases at presentation and there was a similar incidence of bone metastases. Talbot et al. (1980)[49] showed that the probability of liver metastases related to evidence of venous invasion in the operative specimen. Davies and Newlands (1983)[50] proposed a classification which largely retained Dukes' classification but allowed for local excision by adding additional categories and retaining the D category for the case deemed to be beyond the confines of surgery at operation.

Moriya et al. (1989)[51] have pointed out that whilst upward spread in rectal tumours is common and downward spread rare, lateral spread to the internal iliac nodes is commoner than previously thought. They record an 18% internal iliac node involvement in rectal tumours at or below the peritoneal reflection. Lateral node involvement is rare without evidence of inferior mesenteric node metastasis.

Dukes (1937)[52] looked at other aspects of pathology which bear on prognosis namely the grading of the tumour and found that whilst most tumours are moderately well differentiated and show little tendency to submucosal spread, the much rarer poorly differentiated or high-grade tumours showed a greater propensity to submucosal spread. Jass et al. (1987)[53] looked at other variables such as lymphocytic infiltration and the character of the edge of the tumour and confirmed that lymphocytic infiltration was of good prognostic significance whilst an infiltrative edge was of bad prognostic significance and on the basis of this proposed a new system of classification. In the last few years there have been, as yet unsuccessful, international attempts to standardise classification (Jass, 1987)[54]. The consensus conference of the American National Institutes of Health in April 1990 has recommended that the TNM system of classification be adopted for colon and rectal cancer (Hermanek and Sobin, 1987)[55].

One of the key areas in assessing prognosis is analysis of excised lymph nodes. Cawthorn et al. (1986)[56] believe that the yield of lymph nodes is improved by xylose clearance of mesenteric fat. More recently, epithelial markers have been produced which allow the recognition of small numbers of malignant cells in lymph nodes. These are called micrometastases, but their prognostic significance is still uncertain (Cutait et al., 1991)[57].

## Prevention

Primary prevention in colorectal cancer is difficult because there is no agreement as to the cause of colorectal tumours so that educational programmes are difficult to target. Muto et al. (1975)[58] showed that most adenomas grow slowly with a low risk of malignant transformation over a 5–15 year span. The prevalence of adenomas increases with age so that a majority of the population have adenomas by the age of 70 years (Knight et al., 1989)[59]. Screening may be directed to populations above a stipulated age to find and eradicate adenomas or "early" carcinomas by colonoscopy. There is considerable debate as to the cost-effectiveness of this approach (Eddy et al., 1987)[60]. A large population-screening exercise is reported by Hardcastle et al. (1989)[61] in which a random control trial of faecal occult blood assessments has been used to select a group for colonoscopy. They have found adenomas and "earlier" carcinomas in the screened group but have not shown any survival advantage as yet. The difficulties in assessing this type of study with lead time and length time bias are discussed by Heine and Rothenberger (1991)[62]. Screening of high-risk groups such as patients with inflammatory bowel disease, or with a strong family history or patients with previous large bowel tumours, is now accepted as routine (Hardcastle and Thomas, 1989)[63].

## Diagnosis

The clinical assessment of the patient is important. Goulston et al. (1986)[64] reviewed a series of patients over 40 years of age presenting to general practitioners with rectal bleeding. More than 10% of these patients had a carcinoma of the large bowel and in the majority of these patients the general practitioner had believed there was an anal source of bleeding rather than bleeding from the large bowel.

There is no doubt that either colonoscopy or double contrast barium enema (DCBE) plus flexible sigmoidoscopy (FS), in expert hands, have a high sensitivity in the diagnosis of large bowel cancer (Irvine et al., 1988)[65]. Confrontational debate about the merits of the techniques is sterile (Simpkins, 1990)[66]. Hence it is important to see the shortcomings of both investigations. Fork (1988)[67] reviewed radiographic features in patients in whom a colonic carcinoma had been overlooked at barium enema. Retrospectively, all the failures were due to perceptive errors by the radiologist. Glick et al. (1989)[68] reported on 18 lesions greater than 2 cm which were not diagnosed at colonoscopy but were found at DCBE. Rex et al. (1990)[69] compared the diagnostic efficiency of colonoscopy with DCBE plus FS. They found no significant difference in diagnostic yield except that colonoscopy found more small polyps of less than 1 cm. The major advantage of colonoscopy is greater sensitivity in detecting small polyps and allowing biopsy or excision of lesions as appropriate. The defect is that most small polyps are clinically unimportant (Waye, 1988)[70].

There is a small risk of perforation or significant bleeding after polyp removal (Nivatvongs, 1987)[71]. Small perforations without signs of spreading peritonitis have been successfully managed conservatively (Carpio et al., 1989)[72]. What is important is that the whole of the large bowel should be examined before surgery if this is possible because the presence of multiple tumours may alter the strategy of treatment (Isabel-Martinez et al., 1988)[73]. If the whole large bowel cannot be examined before operation it should be assessed, not only at operation, but by colonoscopy (or barium study) within 3 months of the operation. In fact, Tate et al. (1988)[74] recommend postoperative assessment because of the unreliability of preoperative colonoscopy or barium enema. Stewart et al. (1984)[75] showed the value of water-soluble contrast enema to investigate the differential diagnosis between true obstruction and pseudo-obstruction.

It is clear that the extent of local spread and distant metastases are important determinants of survival. In carcinoma of the rectum the accuracy of local palpation has been shown to be high in experienced hands (Nicholls et al., 1982)[76]. Pelvic computed tomography (CT) may refine this a little (Zheng et al., 1984)[77] but endorectal ultrasound has proved very accurate in assessment in expert hands (Glaser et al., 1990)[78]. Endorectal ultrasonography is particularly useful in assessing the depth of penetration in relatively early rectal tumours (Di Candio et al., 1987)[79]. The local assessment of rectal tumours has been the subject of many papers comparing the merits of anorectal ultrasound, CT scanning and nuclear magnetic resonance imaging (MRI). Krestin et al. (1988)[80] compared MRI to CT in the pelvis and believe that the former is more accurate. However, Guinet et al. (1990)[81] conclude that MRI offers no advantage over CT.

Schreve et al. (1984)[82] compared various methods of assessing the liver for metastases. Biochemical tests of liver function had low sensitivity but a high specificity. Isotope scans with technetium, ultrasound scan (US) and computed tomography (CT) had accuracy at 79%–88% with no significant difference between CT and US. Yamaguchi et al. (1991)[83] compared US, CT, hepatic angiography and arterial portography plus CT. They report the superiority of this latter combined technique especially in the detection of deposits smaller than 1 cm. Machi et al. (1987)[84] leave us in no doubt that intraoperative ultrasound is the most sensitive and accurate technique since they report an accuracy of 98%.

Lange and Martin (1991)[85] review the use of radiolabelled, monoclonal antibodies for the detection and demarcation of colorectal tumours. External imaging has proved useful demonstrating recurrence. Intraoperative probes can map the tumour and determine surgical margins.

# Treatment

## Carcinoma Rectum

Radical resection is required for cure in carcinoma rectum in most patients. Heald et al. (1982)[86] emphasised the importance of removing the mesorectum. Quirke et al. (1986)[87] have documented the importance of the lateral margins. Hojo et al. (1989)[88] report that extended lateral dissection significantly improves survival but at the price of increased bladder and sexual dysfunction.

The realisation that longitudinal spread is very limited in most rectal tumours (Williams et al., 1983)[89] has increased the number of patients treated by anterior resection and decreased the number treated by abdominoperineal resection (Kirwan et al., 1989)[90]. Karanjia et al. (1990)[91] have suggested that a margin of 1 cm below the tumour is adequate. The other factor which has increased the anterior resection rate is the use of circular stapling devices (Waxman, 1983)[92].

Small rectal carcinomas which have not penetrated the wall can be adequately treated by local excision with satisfactory results (Graham et al., 1990)[93]. Endocavity radiation is effective in small tumours (Papillon, 1975)[94]. It should be emphasised that this is a very small proportion of patients. Berry et al. (1990)[95] have demonstrated that there is a place for local resection with a resectoscope in the elderly and unfit and in the incurable situation. Brunetaud et al. (1989)[96] summarise a large experience in the use of YAG laser to palliate advanced rectal cancer in an important addition to the growing number of reports of this method.

In rectal cancer, radiotherapy has been used in the preoperative period and has been shown to reduce local recurrence but has little impact on survival (Metzger, 1991)[97]. Preoperative radiotherapy has been shown to be useful in the fixed rectal tumour allowing some of these tumours to become removable (James and Schofield, 1985)[98]. Postoperative radiotherapy has the merit that it allows a selective policy after full histopathology but it carries the risk of radiation injury to the small bowel. The pre- and postoperative studies are reviewed by Metzger and none shows survival benefit.

## Carcinoma Colon

Small colonic tumours with foci of malignancy are being increasingly removed colonoscopically. Christie (1988)[99] reviews the literature and reports on his own experience. Williams et al. (1987)[100] give the criteria for this form of treatment and give encouraging 5-year results.

In carcinoma of the colon, a radical resection with lymph node clearance is required in most patients. Some have suggested that in the young patient or the patient with multiple tumours a total colectomy is the treatment of choice. Turnbull et al. (1967)[101] emphasised vascular and lymphatic disconnection as the first step in the no-touch technique but although they reported improved survival, others have not been able to reproduce this. Surtees et al. (1990)[102] in a good study of high vascular ligation has not been able to show any benefit from this technique.

About 20% of patients with colonic carcinoma present with obstruction (Phillips et al., 1985)[103]. Right-sided lesions have been treated by resection and primary anastomosis for many years but there is an increasing tendency to deal with left-sided obstruction in this fashion. Stephenson et al. (1990)[104] report superior results after subtotal colectomy with primary anastomosis when compared with staged resection in left-colonic obstruction. Radical segmental resection and anastomosis can be effected if the obstructed colon is decompressed and washed clean by the method suggested by the group at St. Mary's (Radcliffe and Dudley, 1983)[105]. Koruth et al. (1985)[106] have reported a low mortality when using this technique to facilitate a primary anastomosis. Many surgeons deal with obstruction in the sigmoid colon by radical resection and delayed anastomosis, the so-called Hartmann's procedure. In locally advanced tumours, excision of the abdominal wall, uterus, bladder fundus or small bowel may allow a radical excision and adds little to the magnitude of the operation (Jeekal, 1987)[107]. Corman (1991)[108] reviews treatment and in the totally irremovable tumour stresses that bypass should be considered and that a stoma is the last resort.

In colonic cancer it has been shown that 5-FU will produce growth restraint in some tumours (Moertel, 1978)[109]. However, individual reports of the use of 5-FU as an adjuvant to surgery have not produced any consistent improvement in survival but a meta-analysis of the acceptable adjuvant trials of 5-FU suggest the possibility of a marginal survival advantage of 3.4% (Buyse et al., 1988)[110]. Recently a regime of levamisole and 5-FU given for 1 year after surgery appears to have produced improved survival in Dukes' C cases (Moertel et al., 1990)[111].

Guillou (1991)[112] reviews the possibilities of immunotherapy for cancer which may have a significant place in the future, particularly with the development of recombinant cytokines such as interferon. However, he points out that enthusiasm for cancer immunotherapy has waxed and waned for half a century so more evidence is required in this field.

## Complications after Surgery

Goligher (1984)[113] describes in some detail the complications which may arise after surgery for colorectal cancer. The important immediate complications are anastomotic dehiscence and infection (wound or intraperitoneal). Those which become apparent shortly after the operation are altered bowel function and urinary and/or sexual difficulties. The principal late complication is recurrent disease which may be local, distant or both.

## Immediate Complications

Goligher et al. (1977)[114] introduced the assessment of colorectal anastomoses by contrast studies and showed that minor subclinical leakage from anastomoses was more common than had previously been supposed, particularly after low anterior resection. Fielding et al. (1980)[115] suggest that the exact technique of anastomosis is unimportant provided it is competently performed. Aldridge et al. (1986)[116] report a multicentre study of 2648 patients, 11% of whom had a clinical leak from their anastomosis and this rose to 25% in anterior resection. The same group have indicated that there is a wide difference in leak rate between different surgeons. Matheson and Irving (1975)[117] reported a 5% leak rate after anterior resection which low figure they ascribe to a meticulous single-layer suture technique which does not include the mucosa.

Aldridge et al. (1986)[116], reporting on colorectal surgery in the late 1970s, record a 25% wound infection rate. Wound and intraperitoneal infection have been dramatically reduced in the last few years. Menaker (1987)[118] stresses minimising contamination and having adequate blood and tissue levels of appropriate antibiotics. There are many studies on various antibiotic combinations but Juul et al. (1987)[119] confirm that a combination of antibiotics giving a wide spectrum of cover for both Gram-positive and Gram-negative organisms gives adequate protection even if given only for a short time intraoperatively. The difficulties inherent in assessing many of the antibiotic trials published are highlighted by Evans and Pollock (1987)[120]. Krukowski and Matheson (1983)[121] reported their experience in the use of tetracycline lavage in a concentration of one gram per litre which they indicated had been important in controlling and reducing infective complications. Hancock (1990)[122] combined tetracycline lavage at the time of surgery with an adequate intraoperative antibiotic regime of metronidazole and a cephalosporin and reports a wound infection rate of about 1% after colorectal surgery.

## Early Complications

Pedersen et al. (1986)[123] showed that the altered bowel habit with low volume stools, urgency and possible incontinence which may occur after low anterior resection is due to less compliance in the anastomosed rectum. Horgan et al. (1989)[124] showed some diminution in internal sphincter resting pressure after very low anastomoses but no change in the external sphincter or the nerve supply. It was considered that this might be due to direct injury to the sphincter. As time passes, the frequency and urgency of defaecation reduces as the compliance increases.

May (1966)[125] reported sexual dysfunction in the form of impotence in male patients after rectal excision. Metcalf et al. (1986)[126] showed that sexual dysfunction also occurred after rectal excision in women. Yaeger and Van Heerden (1980)[127] reported an incidence of 20% in patients having excision for benign disease and even higher figures for rectal excision for malignant disease. Aboseif et al. (1990)[128], with the knowledge that these sexual problems are due to denervation, reviewed the neuroanatomy of the autonomic nerves within the pelvis. It is known that erection requires intact parasympathetic innervation and that ejaculation in the male requires intact sympathetic innervation. Leicester et al. (1984)[129] describe the operative technique of intersphincteric proctectomy which preserves the nerves in inflammatory disease. Unfortunately, more radical surgery is required in malignant disease. Hojo et al. (1991)[130], who carry out very radical surgery for rectal tumours, have described the surgical anatomy of the autonomic pelvic nerves and the technique for their preservation.

Watson and Williams (1952)[131] described the urological complications which occur after excision of the rectum. Bladder dysfunction after pelvic surgery may be due to concomitant bladder neck obstruction but may be due to the development of a neurogenic bladder. Fowler et al. (1978)[132] showed that parasympathetic denervation of the bladder may occur during rectal excision due to autonomic nerve injury leading to a neurogenic bladder. Mundy (1982)[133] suggested that the commonest site of injury during mobilisation of the rectum was at the level of the lateral ligaments. The surgical anatomy previously described in relationship to sexual dysfunction is equally pertinent to the avoidance of the complication of bladder dysfunction.

## Recurrent Tumour and Follow-up Policy

Goligher (1984)[113] sets out two reasons for follow-up of patients after surgery for colorectal cancer. The first of these is for the surgeon's personal audit but the second is to detect recurrence at a stage when further treatment may be helpful. Cochrane et al. (1980)[134] showed that ordinary clinical review very rarely achieved this second objective. Most patients returned with symptomatic recurrence between formal review appointments and it was rare that any effective treatment was possible. Hulton and Hargreaves (1989)[135] represent the view of a number of surgeons when they make the point that simple clinical follow-up of colorectal patients should be abandoned with perhaps more short-term follow-up of high-risk groups. Another response is exemplified by Steele (1986)[136] with much more intensive and frequent follow-up with multiple investigations. Finlay and McArdle (1982)[137] showed that frequent imaging of the liver at an early stage could reveal the presence of occult secondaries. The majority of these were widespread and defined a bad prognosis group but did raise the possibility of early diagnosis of solitary metastases. Colonoscopy, at intervals, in order to eliminate adenomas and prevent or detect metachronous tumours is now accepted by many (Nava and Pagana, 1982)[138]. The principal unresolved problem is whether early detection of local recurrence gives therapeutic advantage. Gilbertsen and Wangensteen (1962)[139] reported the experience of a policy of so-called second look laparotomy, which Dr Wangensteen had introduced 13 years previously. In this the patient, even if asymptomatic, was submitted to a second operation at 6 months to search for residual or recurrent tumour and had laparotomies every 6 months until either tumour-free or inoperably recurrent. They reported a 12% salvage rate but most surgeons felt this was too intrusive and impracticable a policy. The idea was revived by the possibility of markers giving presymptomatic indication of recurrence. Gold and Freeman (1965)[140] described carcinoembryonic antigen (CEA), a reawakened foetal antigen, which was increased in patients with carcinoma of the colon. It was shown subsequently to be increased in other conditions but it has been used extensively as a marker of possible recurrence. Sandler et al. (1984)[141] reviewed various studies of CEA-directed second look laparotomy. In these a laparotomy was carried out if there was a sustained increase in the serum level of CEA and investigation had excluded disease outside the confines of surgery. All the studies show a significant number of negative laparotomies. The yield in increased survival varies in these series but even the best results give only a marginal improvement. Pollard et al. (1989)[142] leave us in no doubt that many local recurrences are untreatable and there is a poor yield in terms of cure even when the lesion is resected. However, worthwhile palliation can be achieved in some patients.

The principal thrust of follow-up should be exclusion of synchronous or metachronous tumours and the early indentification of solitary liver or lung metastases. Hughes et al. (1988)[143] reported a multicentre study in which patients with metachronous metastases largely confined to one lobe of the liver had approximately a 25% 5-year disease-free survival. It has to be emphasised that this applies to less than a quarter of patients with liver metastases. Wilking et al. (1985)[144] report similar satisfactory results in lobectomy or other resection of apparently solitary lung metastasis.

Phillips et al. (1984)[145] pointed out that there is a wide difference in local recurrence rates between individual surgeons. Local recurrence could exceed 30% after low anterior resection, yet Heald and Ryall (1986) report less than 5% local recurrence rate. The reason for these wide variations is discussed by Isbister (1990)[146]. It is apparent that differences must, in some part, be related to surgical technique and adequacy of excision but perhaps some of the difference depends on the selection of the patients and the biological nature of the tumours included in the study.

## References


1. Boyle P, Zaridze DG, Smans M (1985) Descriptive epidemiology of colorectal cancer. Int J Cancer 36:9–18
2. Office of population censuses and surveys (1986) Cancer Survival 1979–1981. Her Majesty's Stationery Office, London
3. Levin KE, Dozois RR (1991) Epidemiology of large bowel cancer. World J Surg 15:562–567
4. Wynder EL, Shigematsu T (1967) Environmental factors in cancer of the colon and rectum. Cancer 20:1520–1561
5. Burkitt DP (1975) Large bowel cancer: an epidemiologic jigsaw puzzle. J Natl Cancer Inst 54:3–6
6. Nigro ND, Singh DV, Campbell RL, Pak MS (1975) Effect of dietary beef fat on intestinal tumor formation by azoxymethane in rats. J Natl Cancer Inst 54:439–442
7. Hill MJ (1975) The role of colonic anaerobes in the metabolism of bile acids and steroids and its relation to colon cancer. Cancer 36:2387–2400
8. Wargovich MJ, Baer AR, Hu PJ, Sumiyoshi H (1988) Dietary factors and colorectal cancer. Gastroenterol Clin North Am 17:727–745

9. Muto T, Bussey HJR, Morson BC (1975) The evolution of cancer of the colon and rectum. Cancer 36:2251–2263
10. Eide TJ (1986) Prevalence and morphological features of adenomas of the large intestine in individuals with and without colorectal carcinoma. Histopathology 10:111–118
11. Bussey HJR, Wallace MH, Morson BC (1967) Metachronous carcinoma of the large intestine and intestinal polyps. Proc R Soc Med 60:208–210
12. Heald RJ, Lockhart-Mummery HE (1972) The lesion of the second cancer of the large bowel. Br J Surg 59:16–19
13. Ekelund G, Lindström CG (1974) Histopathological analysis of benign polyps in patients with carcinoma of the colon and rectum. Gut 15:654–663
14. Correa P (1978) Epidemiology of polyps and cancer. In: Pathogenesis of colorectal cancer. B.C. Morson (ed). Saunders, Philadelphia, pp 126–152
15. Clark JC, Collan Y, Eide TJ et al. (1985) Prevalence of polyps in an autopsy series from areas with varying incidence of large bowel cancer. Int J Cancer 36:179–186
16. Goh HS, Jass JR (1986) DNA content and the adenoma–carcinoma sequence in the colorectum. J Clin Pathol 39:387–392
17. Gilbertsen VA, Nelms JM (1978) Prevention of invasive cancer of the rectum. Cancer 41:1137–1139
18. Lynch HT, Watson P, Lanspa SJ et al. (1988) Natural history of colorectal cancer in hereditary non-polyposis colorectal cancer (Lynch syndromes I and II). Dis Colon Rectum 31:439–444
19. Hordijk ML, Shivananda S (1989) Risk of cancer in inflammatory bowel disease: why are the results in the reviewed literature so varied? Scand J Gastroenterol 170 (Suppl):70–74
20. Sugita A, Sachar DB, Bodian C, Ribeiro MB, Aufses AH, Greenstein AJ (1991) Colorectal cancer in ulcerative colitis. Influence of anatomical extent and age at onset on colitis–cancer interval. Gut 32:167–169
21. Gyde S (1991) Screening for colorectal cancer in ulcerative colitis: dubious benefit and high cost. Gut 31:1089–1091
22. Greenstein AJ, Sachar DB, Smith H, Janowitz HD, Aufses AH (1981) A comparison of cancer risk in Crohn's disease and ulcerative colitis. Cancer 48:2742–2745
23. Mecklin JP (1987) Frequency of hereditary colorectal carcinoma. Gastroenterology 93:1021–1025
24. Gardner EJ (1951) A genetic and clinical study of intestinal polyposis, a predisposing factor for carcinoma of the colon and rectum. Am J Hum Genet 3:167–176
25. Gardner EJ (1962) Follow-up study of a family group exhibiting dominant inheritance for a syndrome including intestinal polyps, osteomas, fibromas and epidermal cysts. Am J Hum Genet 14:376–390
26. Smith WG (1958) Gardner's syndrome and desmoid tumors. Dis Colon Rectum 1:323–332
27. Turcot J, Despres JP, St Pierre F (1959) Malignant tumours of the central nervous system associated with familial polyposis of the colon. Dis Colon Rectum 2:465–468
28. Alm T, Licznerski G (1973) The intestinal polyposes. Clin Gastroenterol 2:577–602
29. Van Stolk R, Sivak MV, Petrini JL et al. (1987) Endoscopic management of upper gastrointestinal polyps and periampullary lesions in familial adenomatous polyposis and Gardner's syndrome. Endoscopy 19:19–22
30. Jagelman DG, DeCosse JJ, Bussey HJR (1988) Upper gastrointestinal cancer in familial adenomatous polyposis. Lancet i:1149–1150
31. Diaz-Lopez M, Menezo JL (1987) Congenital hypertrophy of the retinal pigment epithelium and familial polyposis of the colon. Am J Ophthalmol 103:235–236
32. Herrera L (ed) (1989) Familial adenomatous polyposis. Wiley-Liss, New York
33. Bodmer WF, Bailey CJ, Bussey HJR et al. (1987) Localisation of the gene for familial adenomatous polyposis on chromosome 5. Nature 328:614–616
34. Vogelstein B, Fearon ER, Hamilton SR et al. (1988) Genetic alterations during colorectal tumor development. N Eng J Med 319:525–532
35. Fearon ER, Vogelstein B (1990) A genetic model for colorectal tumorogenesis. Cell 61:759–767
36. Fearon ER, Cho KR, Nigro JM et al. (1990) Identification of a chromosome 18q gene that is altered in colorectal cancer. Science 247:49–50
37. Schofield PF, Walsh S, Tweedle DEF (1986) Survival after treatment of carcinoma of the rectum. Br Med J 293:496–497

38. Cunliffe WJ, Hasleton PS, Tweedle DEF, Schofield PF (1984) Incidence of synchronous and metachronous colorectal carcinoma. Br J Surg 71:941–943
39. Isler JT, Brown PC, Lewis FG, Billingham RP (1987) The role of preoperative colonoscopy in colorectal cancer. Dis Colon Rectum 30:435–439
40. Miles WE (1910) Removal of the rectum for cancer: statistical report on 120 cases. Ann Surg 51:854–862
41. Dukes CE (1930) Spread of cancer of the rectum. Br J Surg 17:643–659
42. Dukes CE (1940) Cancer of the rectum. An analysis of 1000 cases. J Pathol Bacteriol 50:527–539
43. Dukes CE (1945) Discussion on the pathology and treatment of carcinoma of the colon. Proc R Soc Med 38:377–384
44. Kirklin JW, Dockerty MB, Waugh JM (1949) The role of the peritoneal reflection in the prognosis of carcinoma of the rectum and sigmoid colon. Sug Gynecol Obstet 88:326–331
45. Astler VB, Coller FA (1954) The prognostic significance of direct extension of carcinoma of the colon and rectum. Ann Surg 139:846–852
46. Turnbull RB Jr, Kyle K, Watson FR, Spratt J (1967) Cancer of the colon: the influence of no-touch isolation technic on survival rates. Ann Surg 166:420–425
47. Cedermark BJ, Schultz SS, Bakshi S et al. (1977) The value of liver scan in the follow-up study of patients with adenocarcinoma of the colon and rectum. Surg Gynecol Obstet 144:745–748
48. Bacon HE, Jackson CC (1953) Visceral metastases from carcinoma of the distal colon and rectum. Surgery 33:495–505
49. Talbot IC, Ritchie S, Leighton MH et al. (1980) The clinical significance of invasion of veins by rectal cancer. Br J Surg 67:439–442
50. Davies NC, Newlands RC (1983) Terminology and classification of colorectal adenocarcinoma: the Australian clinico-pathological staging system. Aust NZ J Surg 53:211–221
51. Moriya Y, Hojo K, Sawada T, Koyama Y (1989) Significance of lateral node dissection from advanced rectal carcinoma at or below the peritoneal reflection. Dis Colon Rectum 32:307–315
52. Dukes CE (1937) Histological grading of rectal cancer. Proc R Soc Med 30:371–376
53. Jass JR, Love SB, Northover JM (1987) A new prognostic classification of rectal cancer. Lancet i:1303–1306
54. Jass JR (1987) Staging of colorectal cancer (symposium). Int J Colorect Dis ii:123–128
55. Hermanek P Sobin LH (1987) International Union against Cancer: UICC, TNM, classification of malignant tumour, 4th edn. Springer, Berlin, Heidelberg, New York
56. Cawthorn SJ, Gibbs NM, Marks CG (1986) Clearance techniques for the detection of lymph nodes in colorectal cancer. Br J Surg 73:58–60
57. Cutait R, Alves VAF, Lopes LC et al. (1991) Restaging of colorectal cancer based on the identification of lymph node micrometastases through immunoperoxidase staining of CEA and cytokeratins. Dis Colon Rectum 34:917–920
58. Muto T, Bussey HJR, Morson BC (1975) The evolution of cancer of the colon and rectum. Cancer 36:2251–2270
59. Knight KK, Fielding JE, Battista RN (1989) Occult blood screening for colorectal cancer. JAMA 261:587–593
60. Eddy DM, Nugent FW, Eddy JF et al. (1987) Screening for colorectal cancer in a high-risk population: results of a mathematical model. Gastroenterology 92:682–692
61. Hardcastle JD, Chamberlain J, Sheffield J et al. (1989) Randomised controlled trial of faecal occult blood screening for colorectal cancer – results of the first 107 349 subjects. Lancet i:1160–1164.
62. Heine JA, Rothenberger DA (1991) Cost-effective management of colon and rectal cancer. World J Surg 15:597–604
63. Hardcastle JD, Thomas WM (1989) Screening an asymptomatic population for colorectal cancer. In: Clinical gastroenterology: colorectal cancer. N. Mortensen (ed). Baillière-Tindall, London, pp 543–566
64. Goulston KJ, Cook HI, Dent OF (1986) How important is rectal bleeding in the diagnosis of bowel cancer and polyps? Lancet ii:261–264
65. Irvine EJ, O'Connor J, Frost RA et al. (1988) Prospective comparison of double contrast barium enema plus flexible sigmoidoscopy versus colonoscopy in rectal bleeding. Gut 29:1188–1193
66. Simpkins KC (1990) Radiology. Curr Opin Gastroenterol 6:50–53

67. Fork FT (1988) Radiographic findings in overlooked colon carcinomas. A retrospective analysis. Acta Radiologica 29:331–336
68. Glick SN, Teplick SK, Balfe DM et al. (1989) Large colonic neoplasms missed by endoscopy. Am J Radiol 152:513–517
69. Rex DK, Weddle RA, Lehman GA et al. (1990) Flexible sigmoidoscopy plus air contrast barium enema versus colonoscopy for suspected lower gastrointestinal bleeding. Gastroenterology 98:855–861
70. Waye JD (1988) Hyperplastic colon polyps – are they markers? Ann Intern Med 109:851–852
71. Nivatvongs S (1987) Complications in colonoscopic polypectomy: an experience with 1555 polypectomies. Dis Colon Rectum 29:825–830
72. Carpio G, Alber E, Gumbs MA, Gerst PH (1989) Management of colonic perforation after colonoscopy. Dis Colon Rectum 32:624–626
73. Isabel-Martinez L, Chapman AH, Hall RI (1988) The value of a barium enema in the investigation of patients with rectal carcinoma. Clin Radiol 39:531–533
74. Tate JJT, Rawlinson J, Royle GT, Brunton FJ, Taylor I (1988) Preoperative or postoperative colonic examination for synchronous lesions in colorectal cancer. Br J Surg 75:1016–1018
75. Stewart J, Finan PJ, Courtney DF, Brennan TG (1984) Does a water-soluble contrast enema assist in the management of acute large bowel obstruction? A prospective study of 177 cases. Br J Surg 71:799–801
76. Nicholls RJ, York Mason A, Morson BC, Dixon AK, Fry KI (1982) The clinical staging of rectal cancer. Br J Surg 69:404–409
77. Zheng GL, Eddleston B, Johnson RJ, James RD, Schofield PF (1984) Computed tomography scanning in rectal carcinoma. J R Soc Med 77:915–920
78. Glaser F, Schlag P, Herfarth C (1990) Endorectal untrasonography for the assessment of invasion of rectal tumours and lymph node involvement. Br J Surg 77:883–887
79. Di Candio G, Mosca F, Campatelli A, Cei A, Ferrari M, Basolo F (1987) Endosonographic staging of rectal carcinoma. Gastrointest Radiol 12:289–295
80. Krestin GP, Steinbrich W, Friedman G (1988) Recurrent rectal cancer. Diagnosis with MR imaging versus CT. Radiology 168:307–311
81. Guinet C, Buy JN, Ghossain MA et al. (1990) Comparison of magnetic resonance imaging and computed tomography in the preoperative staging of rectal cancer. Arch Surg 125:385–388
82. Schreve RH, Terpstra OT, Ausema LA, Lameris JS, Seijen AJ, Jeckl J (1984) Detection of liver metastases: a prospective study comparing liver enzymes, scintigraphy, ultrasonography and computed tomography. Br J Surg 71:947–949
83. Yamaguchi A, Ishida T, Nishimura G et al. (1991) Detection by CT during arterial portography of colorectal cancer metastases to liver. Dis Colon Rectum 34:37–40
84. Machi J, Isomoto H, Yamashita Y, Kurohiji T, Shirouzu K, Kakegawa T (1987) Intraoperative ultrasonography in screening for liver metastases from colorectal cancer: comparative accuracy with traditional procedures. Surgery 101:678–684
85. Lange MK, Martin EW (1991) Monoclonal antibodies in imaging and therapy of colorectal cancer. World J Surg 15:617–622
86. Heald RJ, Husband EM, Ryall RDH (1982) The mesorectum in rectal cancer surgery – the clue to pelvic recurrence. Br J Surg 69:613–616
87. Quirke P, Durdey P, Dixon MF, Williams NS (1986) Local recurrence of rectal adenocarcinoma due to inadequate surgical resection: histopathological study of lateral tumour spread and surgical excision. Lancet ii:996–998
88. Hojo K, Sawada T, Moriya Y (1989) An analysis of survival and voiding, sexual function after wide iliopelvic lymphadenectomy in patients with carcinoma of the rectum, compared with conventional lymphadenectomy. Dis Colon Rectum 32:128–133
89. Williams NS, Dixon MF, Johnston D (1983) Reappraisal of the 5 cm rule of distal excision for carcinoma of the rectum: a study of distal intramural spread and of patient survival. Br J Surg 70:150–154
90. Kirwan WO, O'Riordain MG, Waldron R (1989) Declining indications for abdominoperineal resection. Br J Surg 76:1061–1063
91. Karanjia ND, Schache DJ, North WRS, Heald RJ (1990) Close shave in anterior resection. Br J Surg 77:510–512
92. Waxman BP (1983) Large bowel anastomoses. II. The circular staplers. Br J Surg 70:64–67

93. Graham RA, Garnsey L, Jessup JM (1990) Local excision of rectal carcinoma. Am J Surg 160:306–312
94. Papillon J (1975) Intracavity irradiation of early rectal cancer for cure: a review of 186 cases. Cancer 36:696–701
95. Berry AR, Souter RG, Campbell WB, Mortensen NJ McC, Kettlewell MGW (1990) Endoscopic transanal resection of rectal tumours: a preliminary report of its use. Br J Surg 77:134–137
96. Brunetaud JM, Maunoury V, Cochelard D, Boniface B, Cortot A, Paris JC (1989) Endoscopic laser treatment for rectosigmoid villous adenoma: factors affecting the results. Gastroenterology 97:272–277
97. Metzger U (1991) Adjuvant therapy for colorectal carcinoma. World J Surg 15:576–582
98. James RD, Schofield PF (1985) Resection of inoperable rectal cancer following radiotherapy. Br J Surg 72:279–281
99. Christie JP (1988) Polypectomy or colectomy? Management of 106 consecutively encountered colorectal polyps. Am Surg 54:93–99
100. Williams CB, Whiteway JE, Jass JR (1987) Practical aspects of endoscopic management of malignant polyps. Endoscopy 19:31–37
101. Turnbull RB Jr, Kyle K, Watson FR, Spratt J (1967) Cancer of the colon: influence of the no-touch isolation technic on survival rates. Ann Surg 166:420–427
102. Surtees P, Ritchie JK, Phillips RKS (1990) High versus low ligation of the inferior mesenteric artery in rectal cancer. Br J Surg 77:618–621
103. Phillips RKS, Hittinger R, Fry JS, Fielding LP (1985) Malignant large bowel obstruction. Br J Surg 72:296–302
104. Stephenson BM, Shandall AA, Farouk R, Griffith G (1990) Malignant left-sided large bowel obstruction managed by subtotal/total colectomy. Br J Surg 77:1098–1102
105. Radcliffe AG, Dudley HA (1983) Intraoperative antegrade irrigation of the large intestine. Surg Gynecol Obstet 156:721–723
106. Koruth NM, Hunter DC, Krukowski ZH, Matheson NA (1985) Immediate resection in emergency large bowel surgery: a 7-year audit. Br J Surg 72:703–707
107. Jeekal J (1987) Can radical surgery influence survival in colorectal cancer? World J Surg 11:412–417
108. Corman ML (1991) Principles of surgical technique in the treatment of carcinoma of the large bowel. World J Surg 15:592–596
109. Moertel CG (1978) Chemotherapy of gastrointestinal cancer. N Engl J Med 229:1049–1052
110. Buyse M, Zelenuich-Jacquotte A, Chalmers TC (1988) Adjuvant therapy of colorectal cancer. JAMA 259:3571–3578
111. Moertel CG, Fleming TR, MacDonald JS et al. (1990) Levamisole and fluorouracil for adjuvant therapy of resected colon carcinoma. N Engl J Med 322:352–358
112. Guillou PJ (1991) Immunotherapy for cancer. Br J Surg 78:1281–1282
113. Goligher JC (1984) Surgery of the anus, rectum and colon, 5th edn. Baillière Tindall, London.
114. Goligher JC, Lee PWR, Simpkins KC, Lintott DJ (1977) A controlled comparison of 1 and 2 layer techniques of suture for high and low colorectal anastomoses. Br J Surg 64:609–614
115. Fielding LP, Stewart-Brown S, Blesovsky L, Keaney G (1980) Anastomotic integrity after operations for large-bowel cancer: a multi-centre study. Br Med J ii:411–414
116. Aldridge MC, Phillips RKS, Hittinger R, Fry JS, Fielding LP (1986) Influence of tumour site on presentation, management and subsequent outcome in large bowel cancer. Br J Surg 73:663–670
117. Matheson NA, Irving AD (1975) Single layer anastomosis after rectosigmoid resection. Br J Surg 62:239–242
118. Menaker GJ (1987) The use of antibiotics in surgical treatment of the colon. Surg Gynecol Obstet 164:581–586
119. Juul P, Claaborg KE, Kronborg O (1987) Single or multiple doses of metronidazole and ampicillin in elective colorectal surgery. Dis Colon Rectum 30:526–528
120. Evans M, Pollock AV (1987) The inadequacy of published random control trials of antibacterial prophylaxis in colorectal surgery. Dis Colon Rectum 30:743–746
121. Krukowski ZH, Matheson NA (1983) The management of peritoneal and parietal contamination in abdominal surgery. Br J Surg 70:440–441
122. Hancock BD (1990) Audit of major colorectal and biliary surgery to reduce the rates of wound infection. Br Med J 301:911–912

123. Pedersen IBK, Christiansen J, Hint K, Jensen P, Olsen J, Mortensen PE (1986) Anorectal function after low anterior resection for carcinoma. Ann Surg 204:133–135
124. Horgan PG, O'Connell PR, Shinkwin CA, Kirwan WO (1989) Effect of anterior resection on anal sphincter function. Br J Surg 76:783–786
125. May RE (1966) Sexual dysfunction following rectal excision for ulcerative colitis. Br J Surg 53:29–30
126. Metcalf AM, Dozois RR, Kelly KA (1986) Sexual function in women after proctocolectomy. Ann Surg 204:624–627
127. Yaeger ES, Van Heerden JA (1980) Sexual dysfunction following proctocolectomy and abdominoperineal resection. Ann Surg 191:169–170
128. Aboseif SR, Matzel KE, Lue TF (1990) Sexual dysfunction after rectal surgery. Perspect Colon Rectal Surg 3:157
129. Leicester RJ, Ritchie JK, Wadsworth J, Thomson JPS, Hawley PR (1984) Sexual function and perineal wound healing after intersphincteric excision of the rectum for inflammatory bowel disease. Dis Colon Rectum 27:244–248
130. Hojo K, Vernava AM, Sugihara K, Katumata K (1991) Preservation of urine voiding and sexual function after rectal cancer surgery. Dis Colon Rectum 34:532–539
131. Watson PC, Williams DI (1952) The urological complications of excision of the rectum. Br J Surg 40:19–28
132. Fowler JW, Bremner DN, Moffat LEF (1978) The incidences and consequences of damage to the parasympathetic nerve supply to the bladder after abdominoperineal resection of the rectum for carcinoma. Br J Urol 50:95–98
133. Mundy AR (1982) An anatomical explanation for bladder dysfunction following rectal and uterine surgery. Br J Urol 54:501–504
134. Cochrane JP, Williams JT, Faber RG, Slack WW (1980) Value of outpatient follow-up after curative surgery for carcinoma of the large bowel. Br Med J i:593–595
135. Hulton NR, Hargreaves AW (1989) Is long-term follow-up of all colorectal cancers necessary? J R Coll Surg Edinb 34:21–24
136. Steele G (1986) Follow-up plans after curative resection of primary colon or rectum cancer. In: Colorectal cancer. G.Steele, R.T Osteen (eds). Marcel Dekker, New York, pp 247–279
137. Finlay IG, McArdle CS (1982) The identification of patients at high risk following curative resection for colorectal carcinoma. Br J Surg 69:583–584
138. Nava H, Pagana TJ (1982) Postoperative surveillance of colorectal cancer. Cancer 49:1043–1047
139. Gilbertsen VA, Wangensteen OH (1962) A summary of 13 years' experience with the second look program. Surg Gynecol Obstet 114:438–442
140. Gold P, Freeman SO (1965) Demonstration of tumour-specific antigens in human colonic carcinomata by immunological tolerance and absorption techniques. J Exp Med 121:439–466
141. Sandler RS, Freund DA, Herbst CA, Sandler DP (1984) Cost-effectiveness of postoperative CE antigen monitoring in colorectal cancer. Cancer 53:193–198
142. Pollard SG, MacFarlane R, Everett WG (1989) Surgery for recurrent colorectal carcinoma – is it worthwhile? Ann R Coll Surg Engl 71:293–298
143. Hughes KS, Rosenstein RB, Songhorabodi S et al. (1988) Resection of the liver for colorectal carcinoma metastases: a multi-institutional study of long-term survivors. Dis Colon Rectum 31:1–4
144. Wilking N, Petrelli NJ, Herrera L, Regal A-M, Millelman A (1985) Surgical resection of pulmonary metastases from colorectal adenocarcinoma. Dis Colon Rectum 28:562–564
145. Phillips RKS, Hittinger R, Blesovsky L, Fry JS, Fielding LP (1984) Local recurrence following "curative" surgery for large bowel cancer. I. The overall picture. II. The rectum and rectosigmoid. Br J Surg 71:12–16, 17–20
146. Isbister WH (1990) Basingstoke revisited. Aust NZ J Surg 63:243

# 13 The Appendix

Smith (1986)[1] has contributed two papers detailing the history of appendicitis. The term acute appendicitis was coined by Fitz (1886)[2] who advised early operation. The condition is common but the incidence appears to be falling in the UK and the United States but is increasing in Africa (Adekunle and Funmilayo, 1986)[3]. Heaton (1987)[4] reviews the possible aetiology; it is felt that obstruction to the appendix predisposes to infection from resident organisms. Lack of dietary fibre with faecolith obstruction has been proposed but it is not supported by recent observations. The hygiene hypothesis suggests that lymphoid hyperplasia due to viral infection causes obstruction leading to appendicitis. Williams and Dixon (1988)[5] suggest that the ova of threadworm (pinworm) are a rare but possible cause of appendicular luminal obstruction. Gilbert et al. (1985)[6] showed that delay in diagnosis led to perforation. They found a perforation rate of 72% in children under 5 years of age with acute appendicitis. Smithy et al. (1986)[7] show diagnostic delay in the aged; patients over 80 years of age had a 92% perforation rate and a high mortality. A third group subject to delay are pregnant women (Horowitz et al., 1985)[8]. The diagnosis of appendicitis has been entirely clinical until recent years (Berry and Malt, 1984)[9]. They point out a dilemma; the surgeon wishes to remove appendixes which are inflamed but this must be timely, i.e. before perforation. They found that the lower the uninflamed appendix rate the higher the perforation rate. They feel that a normal appendicectomy rate has to be accepted as a price to reduce the perforated appendix rate. Hoffmann and Rasmussen (1989)[10] review the investigatory aids for the clinician. They conclude that the white cell count, abdominal radiography, CT scan, peritoneal lavage and isotope imaging have not proved sufficiently reliable and should be discarded. Barium enema is said to be accurate. However, real time ultrasound and the use of a computer data base are the most practical ways of increasing diagnostic accuracy. Laparoscopy will reduce the negative laparotomy rate but is intrusive. Semm (1988)[11] reported on laparoscopic appendicectomy. Scarlett et al. (1986)[12] found that the use of computer-aided diagnosis produced a significant reduction in negative laparotomies coupled with a reduction in appendicular perforation at operation.

The concept of treating an appendix mass conservatively is being challenged by papers such as Hoffmann et al. (1984)[13] who found that 21% failed to settle and 20% had recurrent appendicitis. For many years, right iliac fossa pain was ascribed to chronic or grumbling appendicitis and many normal appendixes were removed with relief of symptoms (Howie, 1968)[14]. Current thinking is that recurring low abdominal pain is usually due to irritable bowel syndrome when appendicectomy will not have any long-term beneficial effect (Heaton,

1984)[15]. However, recurrent appendicitis which benefits from operation is well documented by Crabbe et al. (1986)[16]. Chronic granulomatous inflammation can affect the appendix which in the United States and the United Kingdom is usually due to Crohn's disease (Allen and Biggart, 1983)[17]. If the appendix alone is involved by Crohn's disease it can be safely removed and is adequate treatment (Agha et al., 1987)[18]. In Africa, granulomatous appendicitis is most commonly due to *Schistosoma haematobium* infection (Adebamowo et al. 1991)[19].

The principal problems after appendicectomy are associated with infection. Wound infection and its prevention are analysed by Krukowski et al. (1988)[20]. In a review of the papers published between 1960 and 1985 they conclude that patients can be separated into low-risk and high-risk groups with regard to wound infection. The low-risk group consists of normal and inflamed appendixes without suppuration and the high-risk group consists of gangrenous or perforated appendixes. The use of drains or delayed skin closure is shown to be ineffective in both groups. In the low-risk group a single preoperative or perioperative dose of appropriate antibiotics reduces the wound infection rate. In the high-risk group a therapeutic course of antibiotics covering both aerobic and anaerobic bacteria and starting in the preoperative or perioperative period is required. Operative wound lavage with an antibiotic solution is recommended. Mueller et al. (1986)[21], investigating infertility in women after appendicectomy, found no increase unless there was perforation, when they believe the risk is increased. Dachman et al. (1985)[22] review mucocoele of the appendix and pseudomyxoma peritonei. The mucocoele may be simple with retained secretions secondary to a postinfective stricture or it may be associated with a tumour, cystadenoma or cystadenocarcinoma. Rupture of a mucocoele is one cause of pseudomyxoma peritonei. Sugarbaker et al. (1987)[23] discuss the malignant pseudomyxoma of appendicular and colonic origin.

## Tumours

The appendix may be involved with similar tumours to other areas of the intestine but there are some specific aspects that justify mention. McNeal (1971)[24] states that 85% of appendicular tumours are carcinoids and that they rarely metastasise. Anderson and Wilson (1985)[25] state that the appendix is the commonest site for gastrointestinal carcinoid but there is no report of metastatic spread if the tumour is less than 1 cm in diameter. The patients usually presented as acute appendicitis and carcinoid was found in 0.5% of removed appendixes. Only 2 of 147 patients with appendicular carcinoid had evidence of metastatic spread. They conclude that if a carcinoid is found on histopathology after appendicectomy, right hemicolectomy should only be considered when the tumour is greater than 1.5 cm in diameter.

Schlatter et al. (1987)[26] report that primary carcinoma of the appendix has been reported less than 300 times up to 1985. They describe two types: adenocarcinoma and mucinous cystadenocarcinoma. The latter has a slightly better prognosis. Right hemicolectomy is indicated if there is evidence of invasion. They note that 35% of patients with carcinoma of the appendix have other primary malignancies. Burgess and Done (1989)[27] report that the majority of cases of adenocarcinoma present as acute appendicitis and carcinoma is seen in less than 0.1% of appendicectomies.

# References


1. Smith DC (1986) A historical overview of the recognition of appendicitis. Parts 1 and 2. N Y State J Med 86:571–583, 639–647
2. Fitz RH (1886) Perforating inflammation of the vermiform appendix: with special reference to its early diagnosis and treatment. Am J Med Sci 92:321–346
3. Adekunle OO, Funmilayo JA (1986) Acute appendicitis in Nigeria. J R Coll Surg Edinb 31:102–105
4. Heaton KW (1987) Aetiology of acute appendicitis. Br Med J 294:1632
5. Williams DJ, Dixon MF (1988) Sex, *Enterobius vermicularis* and the appendix. Br J Surg 75:1225–1226
6. Gilbert SR, Emmens RW, Putnam TC (1985) Appendicitis in children. Surg Gynecol Obstet 161:261–265
7. Smithy WB, Wexner SD, Dailey TH (1986) The diagnosis and treatment of acute appendicitis in the aged. Dis Colon Rectum 29:170–173
8. Horowitz MD, Gomez GA, Santiesteban R, Burkett G (1985) Acute appendicitis during pregnancy: diagnosis and management. Arch Surg 120:1362–1367
9. Berry J, Malt RA (1984) Appendicitis near its century. Ann Surg 200:567–575
10. Hoffmann J, Rasmussen O (1989) Aids in the diagnosis of acute appendicitis. Br J Surg 76:774–779
11. Semm K (1988) Die Pelviskopische Appendektomie. Dtsch Med Wochenschr 113:3–5
12. Scarlett PY, Cooke WM, Clarke D, Bates C, Chan M (1986) Computer-aided diagnosis of acute abdominal pain at Middlesborough General Hospital. Ann R Coll Surg Engl 68:179–181
13. Hoffmann J, Lindhard A, Jensen H-E (1984) Appendix mass: conservative management without interval appendicectomy. Am J Surg 148:379–382
14. Howie JGR (1968) The place of appendicectomy in the treatment of young adult patients with possible appendicitis. Lancet i:1365–1367
15. Heaton KW (1984) Irritable bowel syndrome. In: Textbook of gastroenterology. A.D. Bouchier et al. (eds). Baillière Tindall, London
16. Crabbe MM, Norwood SH, Robertson HD, Silva JS (1986) Recurrent and chronic appendicitis. Surg Gynecol Obstet 163:11–13
17. Allen DG, Biggart JD (1983) Granulomatous disease in the vermiform appendix. J Clin Pathol 36:632–638
18. Agha FP, Ghahremani GG, Panella JS, Kaufman MW (1987) Appendicitis as the initial manifestation of Crohn's disease: radiological features and prognosis. AJR 149:515–518
19. Adebamowo CA, Akang EEU, Ladipo JK, Ajao OG (1991) Schistosomiasis of the appendix. Br J Surg 78:1219–1221
20. Krukowski ZH, Irwin ST, Denholm S, Matheson NA (1988) Preventing wound infection after appendicectomy: a review. Br J Surg 75:1023–1033
21. Mueller DA, Daling JR, Moore DE et al. (1986) Appendicectomy and the risk of tubal infertility. N Engl J Med 315:1506–1508
22. Dachman AH, Lichtenstein JE, Friednam AC (1985) Mucocele of the appendix and pseudomyxoma peritonei. Review. AJR 144:923–929
23. Sugarbaker PH, Kern K, Lack E (1987) Malignant pseudomyxoma peritonei of colonic origin. Natural history and presentation of a curative approach to treatment. Dis Colon Rectum 30:772–779
24. McNeal JE (1971) Mechanisms of obstruction in carcinoid tumours of the small intestine. Am J Clin Pathol 56:452–458
25. Anderson JR, Wilson BG (1985) Carcinoid tumours of the appendix. Am J Surg 73:545–546
26. Schlatter MG, McKone T, Scholten DJ, Bonnell BW, De Kryger LL (1987) Primary appendiceal adenocarcinoma. Am Surg 53:434–437
27. Burgess P, Done HJ (1989) Adenocarcinoma of the appendix. J R Soc Med 82:28–29

# 14 Irritable Bowel Syndrome

From the days of Da Costa in 1871[1], the syndrome of irritable bowel has been recognised when he observed "in its essential features it consists of painful and obstinate affection of the intestines in which membranes or skins are voided". Da Costa labelled the condition as membranous enteritis and subsequently found that the chemical analysis of these membranes or skins was in fact mucous. In 1906 Hawkins[2] noted that there was a group of disorders of intestinal function without organic cause which comprised the common form of "constipation, nervous diarrhoea, enteralgia, enterospasm and mucus colic." He stressed that these disorders were not amenable to surgical treatment. In 1928, Ryle[3] observed that abdominal pain unassociated with any demonstrable organic change had been described in the literature as spastic constipation, chronic colospasm, spastic colon and tonic hardening of the colon. He added mucomembranous colitis as part of the spectrum. All these terms are indicative of what we now call the irritable bowel syndrome (IBS). Because of the lack of positive laboratory investigation it is very difficult to judge the percentage of patients suffering from IBS in the general population. It has been estimated that 14% of the "healthy population" have symptoms suggestive of IBS (Thompson and Heaton, 1978)[4]. This figure is greatly increased in patients referred to specialised gastrointestinal units and in fact it is said to be the commonest disorder encountered by gastroenterologists (Harvey et al., 1983)[5]. The majority of patients are women, the sex ratio is approximately 2 : 1. Most authors agree that the prevalence of the disease is greater under the age of 40 (Waller and Misiewicz, 1969)[6].

## Symptoms

The diagnosis of IBS is totally dependent upon clinical criteria (Thompson et al., 1989)[7]. The cardinal symptoms are disturbance of bowel habit with or without abdominal pain and distension. Chaudhary and Truelove (1962)[8] recognised two types of IBS on clinical criteria. They called the commoner "spastic colon" but recognised that 23% of their patients had a painless diarrhoea type of IBS. In the painful variety of IBS, the pain is variable in severity, extent, distribution and periodicity. Manning et al. (1978)[9] laid down six discriminating symptoms for painful IBS which would distinguish the condition from organic bowel disease:

1. Pain relieved by bowel action

2. More frequent stools with the onset of pain
3. Looser stools with the onset of pain
4. Visible abdominal distension
5. Rectal passage of mucus
6. A sensation of incomplete rectal emptying

The more of these symptoms that were present the more likely was the diagnosis of IBS. Talley et al. (1990)[10] investigated these criteria and found them to be reliable especially so in young females. Extracolonic manifestations of irritable bowel syndrome are common and Maxton et al. (1991)[11] have shown that non-colonic symptoms, particularly lethargy and backache, are much commoner in irritable bowel syndrome than in a wide range of organic gastrointestinal diseases they have studied. They emphasise that patients with both upper and lower gastrointestinal symptoms are much more likely to have IBS than organic bowel disease. They list other symptoms found in IBS – abdominal distension, excessive flatulance, nausea, heartburn, urgency of micturition, urinary frequency, bad breath, dyspepsia and dysphagia. Abdominal distension is one of the principal features of IBS (Maxton et al., 1989)[12]. It is characteristically absent in the morning but progressively appears during the day and is exacerbated by eating (Heaton, 1984)[13]. Maxton et al (1991)[14] have shown that the distension is not gaseous but may be related to changes in motility or tone of gastrointestinal smooth muscle. They felt that exaggerated lumbar lordosis and lowering of the diaphragm were not significant.

## Aetiology

The aetiology of IBS is unknown. However, certain factors are thought to precipitate the symptoms or at least to motivate the patient to take his or her symptoms to a doctor for a diagnosis of IBS to be made. Drossman et al. (1988)[15] compares IBS patients with a group of people who have not sought medical treatment but had abdominal symptoms of IBS on questioning. The IBS patients had an excess of abnormal personality patterns and had lesser coping capability. As far back as 1906 Hawkins[2] suggested that the disorder was more in the upper and middle class patients compared with the working class and this was supported by Hardy (1945)[16]. The incidence of the disorder has been thought to be increased at times when life stresses and responsibilities are high (Peters and Bargain, 1944)[17]. Palmer et al. (1974)[18] found that 50% of patients thought their symptoms were related to stress. It was felt that many patients had a moderate degree of psychoneurotic disorder in the form both of neurotic personality structure and presence of psychoneurotic symptoms. Ford et al. (1987)[19] showed that patients with IBS had a greater prevalence of previous or current psychiatric disease than patients with organic bowel disease.

Studies of the motility in IBS have been difficult to interpret. Almy (1951)[20] showed that pressure in the sigmoid colon in normal subjects and in patients with spastic colon was increased by stress while those with painless diarrhoea showed a profound hypomotility. By contrast, Chaudhary and Truelove (1962)[8] ascertained no significant differences in pressure response to stress between normal subjects and patients with irritable bowel syndrome. More recently, studies have concentrated upon myoelectrical potentials in the sigmoid colon. The results suggest that in IBS there is a high incidence of three cycles per minute slow wave activity (Snape et al., 1977)[21]. This pattern is seen in patients with constipation and with diarrhoea and appears to be constant even during asymptomatic phases (Taylor et al., 1978)[22]. Kumar and Wingate (1985)[23] showed that psychological stress induces greater alterations in the motor pattern of patients with IBS than in normal subjects. Frexinos et al. (1987)[24] have shown increased propagated activity in the colon in response to food in patients with the painless diarrhoea type of IBS.

There is evidence of generalised smooth muscle abnormality as demonstrated by oesophageal manometry (Whorwell et al., 1981)[25] and bladder cystometry (Whorwell et al., 1986)[26]. Preston et al. (1985)[27] demonstrated abnormalities in gastrointestinal hormones in IBS which may relate to the altered motor function. Other suggestions as to causation such as abuse of purgatives and the development of the condition after infection have been shown to be separate entities. Similarly, Pena and Truelove (1972)[28] have shown that the condition is not due to lactose malabsorption.

## Treatment

Drossman (1987)[29] states that sympathetic discussion is the most important aspect of treatment. The benign nature of the condition must be stressed as many patients are convinced that they have a serious organic disease. In rare cases more intensive psychotherapy may be required.

In the past, a low-fibre diet was recommended but this has now been changed drastically to a high-fibre diet. Manning et al. (1977)[30] have shown in a controlled trial that a high-fibre diet in IBS improves symptoms and some aspects of colonic motility but a low-fibre diet does not. Lucey et al. (1987)[31] have questioned this after a trial of bran against placebo showed good improvement in both groups. Read (1990)[32] states that IBS is a condition which has been treated with a great variety of drugs without notable success. Antidepressant drugs are useful in patients who show features of depression (Rose et al., 1986)[33]. Whorwell et al. (1987)[34] report on their experience with hypnotherapy in IBS and indicate a high success rate in selected patients with typical symptoms.

## References

1. Da Costa JM (1871) Membranous enteritis. Am J Med Sci 62:321
2. Hawkins HP (1906) The reality of enterospasm and its mimicry of appendicitis. Br Med J i:65–69
3. Ryle JA (1928) Chronic spasmodic affections of the colon and the disease which they stimulate. Lancet ii:1115–1119
4. Thompson WG, Heaton KW (1978) Functional bowel disorder, a new perspective. Gut 19:975

5. Harvey FRD, Salih SY, Read AE (1983) Organic and functional disorders in 2000 gastroenterology outpatients. Lancet i:632–634
6. Waller SL, Misiewicz JJ (1969) Prognosis in the irritable bowel syndrome, prospective study. Lancet ii:753–756
7. Thompson WD, Drossman DA, Dotevall G, Heaton KW, Kruis W (1989) Irritable bowel syndrome: guidelines for the diagnosis. (IBS Working Team report, Rome 1988) Gastroenterology 2:92–95
8. Chaudhary NA, Truelove SC (1962) The irritable bowel colon syndrome; a study of the clinical features, predisposing causes and prognosis in 130 cases. Q J Med 31:307–322
9. Manning AP, Thompson WG, Heaton KW, Morris AF (1978) Towards positive diagnosis of the irritable bowel. Br Med J ii:653–654
10. Talley NJ, Phillips SF, Melton LJ, Mulvihill C, Wiltgen C, Zinsmeister AR (1990) Diagnostic value of the Manning criteria in irritable bowel syndrome. Gut 31:77–81
11. Maxton DG, Morris JA, Whorwell PJ (1991) More accurate diagnosis of irritable bowel syndrome by the use of "non-colonic" symptomatology. Gut 32:784–786
12. Maxton DG, Morris JA, Whorwell PJ (1989) Ranking of symptoms by patients with the irritable bowel syndrome. Br Med J 299:1138
13. Heaton KW (1984) Irritable bowel syndrome. In: Textbook of gastroenterology. A.D. Bouchier et al. (eds). Baillière-Tindall, London, p 867
14. Maxton DG, Martin DF, Whorwell PJ, Godfrey M (1991) Abdominal distension in female patients with irritable bowel syndrome: exploration of possible mechanisms. Gut 32:662–664
15. Drossman DA, McKee DC, Sandler RS et al. (1988) Psychosocial factors in the irritable bowel syndrome. A multivariant study of patients and non-patients with irritable bowel syndrome. Gastroenterology 95:701–708
16. Hardy TL (1945) Order and disorder in the large intestine. Lancet i:519–524
17. Peters GA, Bargain JE (1944) The irritable bowel syndrome. Gastroenterology 3:399–402
18. Palmer RL, Stonehill E, Crisp AH, Walker SL, Misiewicz JJ (1974) Psychological characteristics of patients with irritable bowel syndrome. Postgrad Med J 50:416–469
19. Ford MJ, Miller PM, Eastwood J, Eastwood MA (1987) Life events, psychiatric illness and the irritable bowel syndrome. Gut 28:160–165
20. Almy TP (1951) Experimental studies on irritable colon. Am J Med 10:60–67
21. Snape WJ, Carlson GM, Matarazzo SA, Cohen S (1977) Evidence that abnormal myoelectrical activity produces colonic motor dysfunction in the irritable bowel syndrome. Gastroenterology 72:383–387
22. Taylor I, Darby C, Hammond P (1978) Comparison of rectosigmoid myoelectrical activity in the irritable colon syndrome during relapses and remissions. Gut 19:923–929
23. Kumar D, Wingate DL (1985) The irritable bowel syndrome: a paroxysmal motor disorder. Lancet ii:973–977
24. Frexinos J, Fioramonti J, Bueno I (1987) Colonic myoelectrical activity in IBS painless diarrhoea. Gut 28:1613–1618
25. Whorwell PJ, Clouter C, Smith CL (1981) Oesophageal motility in irritable bowel syndrome. Br Med J 282:1101
26. Whorwell PJ, Lupton EW, Erduran D, Wilson K (1986) Bladder smooth muscle dysfunction in patients with irritable bowel syndrome. Gut 27:1014–1017
27. Preston DM, Adrian TE, Christofides N-D et al. (1985) Positive correlation between symptoms and circulating motilin, pancreatic polypeptide and gastrin concentrations in functional bowel disorders. Gut 26:1059–1064
28. Pena AS, Truelove SC (1972) Hypolactasia in irritable colon syndrome. Scand J Gastroenterol 7:433–438
29. Drossman DA (1987) Psychosocial treatment of the refractory patient with irritable bowel syndrome. J Clin Gastroenterol 9:253–255
30. Manning AP, Heaton KW, Harvey RF, Uglow P (1977) Wheat fibre and irritable bowel syndrome. Lancet ii:417
31. Lucey MR, Clark ML, Lowndes J, Dawson AM (1987) Is bran efficacious in irritable bowel syndrome – a double-blind placebo-controlled crossover study. Gut 28:221–225
32. Read NW (1990) Motility: functional diseases. Curr Opin Gastroenterol 6:9–13
33. Rose RD, Traughton AH, Harvey JS, Smith PM (1986) Depression and functional bowel disorders in gastrointestinal out-patients. Gut 27:1025–1028
34. Whorwell PJ, Prior A, Colgan SM (1987) Hypnotherapy in severe irritable bowel syndrome: further experience. Gut 28:423–425

# 15 Diverticular Disease

Diverticular disease most commonly is a disease of ageing. Slack (1962)[1] pointed to the herniation of mucosa through points of weakness in the colonic wall. These weak areas are at the point of entry of the vasa recta en route to supply the mucosa and are between the taeniae coli.

Painter (1964)[2] in a classical paper, emphasised the importance of raised intraluminal pressure leading to pulsion diverticula. Painter and Burkitt (1971)[3] suggested that the generation of the high pressure areas within the colon were due to the low-residue diet prevalent in Western society. These authors indicated that diverticular disease was virtually unknown in many parts of Africa where the diet is high in fibre.

There are many studies reviewing both autopsy material and radiological studies which show a high incidence of diverticular disease increasing with age with particular prevalence after the seventh decade. A study in Northern Ireland showed that half the population over the age of 80 have diverticular disease (Parks, 1968)[4].

Any symptoms associated with uncomplicated diverticular disease are due to spasm of the bowel, not the diverticula themselves (Thompson, 1986)[5]. Problems with diverticular disease occur because of complications (diverticulitis, fistula formation, obstruction or haemorrhage). The other significant factor in diverticular disease is that it may coexist with Crohn's disease or carcinoma which increases the difficulty of diagnosis (McCue et al., 1989)[6].

## Pathology

Morson (1963)[7] noted considerable muscle thickening due to hypertrophy and suggested that this predated the development of the diverticula. The hypertrophied circular muscle raises transverse folds in the mucosa and the hypertrophied segment becomes thickened and irregularly contracted with shortening of the segment even in the absence of inflammation. More recently Whiteway and Morson (1985)[8] have shown that there is an increased amount of elastic tissue in the colonic wall in this condition. This was the first description of the ultrastructure of the colonic muscle in diverticular disease. Mucosal laxity is characteristically seen in diverticular disease so that the mucosa in the sigmoid colon may prolapse and become inflamed to produce segmental (or crescentic) colitis (Sladen and Filipe, 1984)[9].

The distribution of the disease was studied by Parks (1969)[10] when he studied almost 500 cases of diverticular disease diagnosed by barium enema. The sigmoid colon was involved alone in two thirds of the cases and was involved in combination with the rest of the colon in almost all the remainder: 4% had right-sided disease alone. This is a typical distribution in Western communities and is to be contrasted with the much higher incidence of right-sided disease revealed in communications based on experience in oriental areas (Lee, 1986)[11]. Graham and Ballantyne (1987)[12] indicated that isolated right-sided diverticular disease appears to occur in younger patients and is more likely to be congenital in origin. The complications of right-sided disease are similar but there seems to be a higher incidence of haemorrhage as compared to inflammation. When a right-colonic diverticulum is inflamed it may simulate appendicitis and at operation can be difficult to distinguish from a carcinoma but a right-colonic resection is an acceptable treatment.

## Complications

Despite the prevalence of diverticular disease, not more that 1%–2% of the population have inflammatory complications and less than half of these require surgery (Kyle and Davidson, 1975)[13]. The incidence of inflammatory complications is increased by the use of steroids or non-steroidal anti-inflammatory drugs (Corda, 1987)[14].

Minor bleeding rarely if ever occurs from diverticular disease but massive bleeding may occur in particular in association with right-sided lesions. Milewski and Schofield (1989)[15] reviewed the topic of massive colonic bleeding and point out the difficulty in distinguishing bleeding from right-sided diverticular disease and right-sided angiodysplasia (vascular ectasia). Boley and Brandt (1986)[16] give a full review of every aspect of angiodysplasia.

## Treatment

In the past there was a tendency to operate more readily in diverticular disease but it is now accepted that surgery should be reserved for the complications. A good review of the medical management of diverticular disease comes from Pohlman (1988)[17]. The diagnostic difficulties between diverticular disease and tumour can occur both as a result of difficulty in radiology and as a result of difficulty in operative assessment (Lambert et al. 1986)[18]. Similar difficulties may be encountered in differentiating between segmental Crohn's disease of the sigmoid colon and diverticulitis (Schmidt et al., 1968)[19]. Indeed, it is not surprising since diverticular disease is so common that coexistent Crohn's disease and diverticulosis may occur in the sigmoid colon (McCue et al., 1989)[6].

## Surgical Treatment

### *Inflammation*

There have been some differences in opinion concerning the indications for operation in septic complications. Many American surgeons would operate after one attack of diverticulitis but their British counterparts would continue conservative treatment if a single attack settled. There have been reports of percutaneous drainage of pericolic abscesses to allow an acute problem to resolve so that elective surgery could be carried out at a later date. Neff et al. (1987)[20] record the successful application of this method. Resection for diverticular disease includes removal of the whole of the sigmoid colon. Benn et al. (1986)[21] in a large review support the view that the anastomosis must be done to the upper rectum. They show a significantly lower recurrence rate when this element of technique has been followed.

If, at presentation, there is evidence of spreading peritonitis or generalised peritonitis there is no doubt that surgery is indicated. The results of an uncontrolled British series (Lambert et al., 1986)[18] would indicate that laparotomy with drainage should be discarded. There was little difference in mortality between a defunctioning colostomy and resection unless there was an obvious perforation in the sigmoid colon when resection was superior. Krukowski et al. (1985)[22] reviewed the literature and showed that resection appeared to be the best option in this situation. Finlay and Carter (1987)[23] confirm that in perforated diverticular disease emergency resection carried a lower morbidity but had not a statistically significant difference in mortality when compared to simple colostomy. Woods et al. (1988)[24] reviewed a large series of internal fistulas due to diverticular disease. The most common fistula was colovesical but one quarter of the cases had colovaginal fistulas. Other internal fistulas were rare. They believe that one-stage resection is the treatment of choice. Rao et al. (1987)[25] came to the same conclusion about treatment. They emphasise that most of these patients present with urinary tract rather than bowel symptoms and that cystoscopy almost always suggests the presence of a fistula.

### *Bleeding*

Attempts to localise bleeding by angiography (Uden et al., 1986)[26] or by vascular isotope tagging (Kester et al., 1984)[27] have been found useful in the hands of some authors but Brearley et al., (1986)[28] did not find localising methods satisfactory. The effectiveness of localising methods probably depends upon a high degree of expertise in individual departments. Milewski and Schofield (1989)[15] confirmed previous observations that massive colonic bleeding almost always came from a right-sided lesion, either diverticular disease or angiodysplasia. They review the literature and put a strong argument for treatment by right hemicolectomy in the majority of cases which come to operation. Others, including Slack (1983)[29], have suggested a subtotal or total colectomy is the treatment of choice.

# References


1. Slack WW (1962) The anatomy, pathology and some clinical features of diverticulitis of the colon. Br J Surg 50:185–196
2. Painter NS (1964) The aetiology of diverticulosis of the colon with special reference to the action of certain drugs on the behaviour of the colon. Ann R Coll Surg Engl 34:98–119
3. Painter ND, Burkitt DP (1971) Diverticular disease of the colon: a deficiency disease of Western civilisation. Br Med J ii:450–454
4. Parks TG (1968) Post-mortem studies on the colon with special reference to diverticular disease. Proc R Soc Med 61:932–934
5. Thompson WG (1986) Do colonic diverticula cause symptoms? Am J Gastroenterol 81:613–614
6. McCue J, Copper MJ, Rasbridge SA, Lock MR (1989) Co-existent Crohn's disease and sigmoid diverticulosis. Postgrad Med J 65:636–639
7. Morson BC (1963) The muscle abnormality in diverticular disease of the sigmoid colon. Br J Radiol 36:385–392
8. Whiteway J, Morson BC (1985) Elastosis in diverticular disease of the sigmoid colon. Gut 26:258–266
9. Sladen GE, Filipe MI (1984) Is segmental colitis a complication of diverticular disease? Dis Colon Rectum 27:513–514
10. Parks TG (1969) Natural history of diverticular disease of the colon. A review of 521 cases. Br Med J iv:639–642
11. Lee Y-S (1986) Diverticular disease of the large bowel in Singapore: an autopsy study. Dis Colon Rectum 29:330–335
12. Graham SM, Ballantyne GH (1987) Cecal diverticulitis: a review of the American experience. Dis Colon Rectum 30:821–826
13. Kyle J, Davidson AI (1975) The changing pattern of hospital admissions for diverticular disease of the colon. Br J Surg 62:537–541
14. Corda A (1987) Steroids, non-steroidal anti-inflammatory drugs and serious septic complications of diverticular disease. Br Med J 295:1238
15. Milewski PJ, Schofield PF (1989) Massive colonic haemorrhage: the case for right hemicolectomy. Ann R Coll Surg Engl 71:253–259
16. Boley SJ, Brandt LJ (1986) Vascular ectasias of the colon. Dig Dis Sci 31:26S–42S
17. Pohlman T (1988) Diverticulitis. Surg Clin North Am 17:357–385
18. Lambert ME, Knox RA, Schofield PF, Hancock BD (1986) Management of the septic complications of diverticular disease. Br J Surg 73:576–579
19. Schmidt GT, Lennard-Jones JE, Morson BC, Young AC (1968) Crohn's disease of the colon and its distinction from diverticulitis. Gut 9:7–16
20. Neff CC, van Sonnerberge E, Casola G et al. (1987) Diverticular abscesses: percutaneous drainage. Radiology 163:15–18
21. Benn PL, Wolff BG, Ilstrup DM (1986) Level of anastomosis and recurrent colonic diverticulitis. Am J Surg 151:269–271
22. Krukowski ZH, Koruth NM, Matheson NA (1985) Evolving practice in acute diverticulitis. Br J Surg 72:684–686
23. Finlay IG, Carter DC (1987) A comparison of emergency resection and staged management in perforated diverticular disease. Dis Colon Rectum 30:929–933
24. Woods RJ, Lavery IC, Fazio VW, Jagelman DG, Weakley FL (1988) Internal fistulas in diverticular disease. Dis Colon Rectum 31:591–596
25. Rao PN, Knox R, Barnard RJ, Schofield PF (1987) Management of colovesical fistula. Br J Surg 74:362–363
26. Uden P, Jiborn H, Jonsson K (1986) Influence of selective mesenteric arteriography on the outcome of emergency surgery for massive low gastrointestinal haemorrhage: a 15-year experience. Dis Colon Rectum 29:561–566
27. Kester RR, Welch JP, Sziklas JP (1984) The $^{99m}$Tc-labelled RBC scan. A diagnostic method for low gastrointestinal bleeding. Dis Colon Rectum 27:47–52
28. Brearley S, Hawker PC, Dorricott NS et al. (1986) The importance of laparotomy in the diagnosis and management of intestinal bleeding of obscure origin. Ann R Coll Surg Engl 68:245–248
29. Slack WW (1983) Surgery for massive haemorrhage from the large intestine. In: Robb and Smith's operative surgery. 3. Colon, rectum and anus, 4th edn. I.P. Todd, L.P. Fielding (eds). Butterworth, London, pp 268–269

# 16 Motility Disorders

A number of conditions lead to severe constipation. Christensen (1971)[1] suggested that motility disorders of the gastrointestinal tract were due to one of three causes: either a defect in smooth muscle of the bowel, a defect in the intrinsic or extrinsic nerve supply or an abnormality of gastrointestinal hormones. The last of these is still ill-understood but hormones secreted by the intestinal neuroendocrine cells affect gastrointestinal motility and the subject is reviewed by Lluis and Thompson (1988)[2]. Lack of other hormones such as in myxoedema is well recognised to be associated with constipation (Abbasi et al., 1975)[3]. It seems appropriate to discuss in some detail diseases caused by apparent or presumed neurological or smooth muscle disorders.

## Hirschsprung's Disease

Dalla Valle (1920)[4] described the disease process in infants with severe constipation and an empty undilated rectum. He noted that there was a familial incidence and that the wall of the rectum contained no ganglion cells. The condition usually presents in the neonate or in early infancy and Eek and Knutrud (1962)[5] noted that without treatment half the children died in the first year of life and very few reached adulthood. Nevertheless, the condition may not present until later in life but there is always a history of constipation going back to early childhood (Todd, 1977)[6].

Swenson and Bill (1948)[7] were the first to publish surgical treatment of this functional obstruction. They noted that the bowel was dilated above an undilated segment and that it was this undilated area which was abnormal due to being aganglionic. Their method of management was to resect the aganglionic segment and carry out an abdominoanal pullthrough. Norberg (1964)[8] noted that the ganglia acted as the final common path for the autonomic influences and in their absence there was uncoordinated contraction leading to functional obstruction. Nixon (1984)[9] states that the length of the disease segment is variable but its distal margin is within 1 to 2 cm of the dentate line. In two thirds of the cases, the aganglionic segment includes the rectum and lower sigmoid colon. The next most common type is described as short segment involving part of the rectum only but others involve greater amounts of colon and, on occasions, may be total colonic. In a very small proportion of cases the aganglionic segment is only 1–2 cm in length. This is referred to as ultra-short segment disease and can be difficult to diagnose.

Nixon (1985)[10] reviews the typical clinical picture, diagnosis and management in children. Fraser and Berry (1967)[11] review the most dangerous complication, enterocolitis, which carries a high mortality, particularly in neonates. Frank and Nixon (1979)[12] showed this to be the cause of death in 56% of patients who die after operation.

Barium enema carried out on the unprepared bowel is a reliable guide to diagnosis and extent of disease, even in the neonatal period (Nixon, 1985)[10]. Swenson and Bill (1948)[7] suggested full thickness biopsy to confirm the absence of ganglion cells. Noblett (1969)[13] has claimed that suction biopsy gives adequate material for histological diagnosis. Lake et al. (1978)[14] have found that examination of a suction biopsy using a histochemical technique to demonstrate acetyl cholinesterase activity is completely error-free in reaching a diagnosis. Lawson and Nixon (1967)[15] showed that the rectoanal reflex is absent even in ultra-short segment disease. In this reflex, balloon dilatation of the rectum produces relaxation of the internal sphincter. Nixon (1985)[10] says that this type of manometry can be misleading in the neonatal period but is especially useful in older children who may have ultra-short segment disease.

In addition to the rectosigmoidectomy described by Swenson and Bill[7], two other procedures have been widely used, the Duhamel retrorectal transanal anastomosis (Duhamel, 1960)[16] and the endorectal technique of Soave (1964)[17]. Nixon (1985)[10] suggests a preliminary colostomy in the neonate and a covering colostomy in older children. Ideally he performs the definitive operation at about 3 months. He compares the three types of procedure and finds they all give satisfactory results in most patients but he favours the Duhamel procedure in long segment disease and states that it gives a better reservoir. Canty (1982)[18] has introduced modifications by the use of the GIA stapler to divide the colorectal septum. Lynn and Van Heerden (1975)[19] showed that extended internal sphincterotomy gives satisfactory results in ultra-short segment disease. A modern review of the disease in children comes from Doig (1991)[20].

There are few series dealing with the disease in adults. McCredy and Beart (1980)[21] analysed 60 cases which had been managed in the Mayo Clinic. All of the three major operative procedures have produced fairly satisfactory results. Elliott and Todd (1985)[22], reviewing the cases at St Mary's Hospital, found the Duhamel procedure much the most satisfactory.

## Chagas' Disease

In South America a type of severe constipation caused by *Trypanosoma cruzi* was recognised by Chagas (1916)[23]. Most patients recover from the acute phase of the disease but then go into the chronic phase characterised by dilatation of the alimentary tract, particularly the oesophagus and colon. Ferreira-Santos (1961)[24] describing his practice in Brazil, said that many of his patients had abnormalities causing both megaoesophagus and megacolon. Köberle and Nador (1956)[25] demonstrated a gross reduction but not an absence of ganglion cells and muscle fibres harbouring the parasite. It was postulated that the inflammatory reaction caused by the organism caused a disturbance of the ganglion cell function. Corrêa Netto et al. (1962)[26] excised the rectum and sigmoid colon and performed a coloanal anastomosis. Haddad (1969)[27] preferred to use the modified Duhamel technique and Habr-Gama et al. (1982)[28] reported excellent results from a series of patients treated by this method. Cutait and Cutait (1991)[29] present a review of management which illustrates the details of operations.

## Idiopathic Constipation

Callaghan and Nixon (1964)[30] described an acquired condition in children with an insensitive but compliant rectum. This has to be distinguished from ultra-short segment Hirschsprung's disease by manometry and biopsy. The rectum is greatly enlarged and the child has persistent soiling but the condition tends to occur only from the second year. Nixon (1984)[9] indicates that with careful persistent medical treatment, many of these cases can be managed satisfactorily. Occasionally, resection of the enlarged rectum is justified.

Idiopathic megarectum and megacolon in adults have been reviewed by Lane and Todd (1977)[31]. They divide this into three groups: megarectum alone, megarectum with colonic dilatation and megacolon alone. The last is unusual. There is no apparent neural abnormality and they showed diminished rectal sensation in many but not all. They found that half of their patients could be managed conservatively with rectal evacuation by manual means and washouts followed by large doses of saline aperients. Surgery is reserved for the failure of medical treatment and is unpredictable. Lane and Todd (1977)[31] found that only 7 of 14 had satisfactory results after subtotal colectomy and caecorectal or ileorectal anastomosis. Read et al. (1985)[32] investigated faecal impaction in the elderly where there is a similar loss of rectal sensitivity and tone leading to an inability to evacuate the rectum. The authors believe this may have a neurological basis and is a difficult management problem.

There are some cases of severe constipation which do not have rectal or colonic dilatation. Routine contrast studies are normal but the patient may go weeks between acts of defaecation. Cummings (1984)[33] explains the basis of medical treatment with increased dietary fibre and bulking agents. In addition to this, stimulant laxatives are used by many physicians. This subject was reviewed by Tedesco and Dipiro (1985)[34]. Bannister et al. (1988)[35] showed that many young women with severe constipation had additional urological abnormalities. Krevsky et al. (1989)[36] confirmed colonic inertia and slow movement within the colon using a radioisotope technique. This supports previous studies done with markers. When medical treatment completely fails, surgery may be considered. Kamm et al. (1988)[37] reported on subtotal colectomy with ileorectal or caecorectal anastomosis in 44 women who had had severe intractable constipation with a normal diameter colon and slow transit. After surgery 50% had a normal bowel function and a majority of the remainder had some diarrhoea. Many of the patients continued to complain of pain but there was poor correlation with preoperative testing.

Orrom et al. (1991)[38] discuss the other pathophysiological cause of chronic colonic constipation, namely obstructed defaecation. They point out that both posterior division of the internal sphincter and lateral division of puborectalis have been disappointing in their effect. They report on rectopexy in patients with obstructed defaecation but this procedure has not produced improvement in most patients' symptoms. These reports are disappointing in the light of Read et al.'s (1986)[39] demonstration of paradoxical puborectalis contraction in patients with outflow obstruction. Kawimbe et al. (1991)[40] review the condition of outflow obstruction. They give a more hopeful report about the use of biofeedback to train individuals to reduce their abnormal pelvic floor EMG activity.

## Visceral Myopathy and Neuropathy

Visceral myopathy and neuropathy are rare conditions which may affect all or part of the gastrointestinal tract. Familial visceral myopathies are a group of diseases in which the smooth muscle of the gut is replaced by fibrous tissue (Mitros et al., 1982)[41]. This leads to dilated segments of the gastrointestinal tract and in some variants the urinary tract is involved. The commonest type involves the oesophagus, duodenum, colon and bladder (Schuffler et al., 1977)[42]. Familial visceral neuropathies are even rarer and show normal smooth muscle but degeneration of the myenteric plexus and appear to affect the small intestine chiefly (Roy et al., 1980)[43]. Chinn and Schuffler (1988)[44] have shown that intestinal pseudo-obstruction due to a neuropathy involving the myenteric plexus may be associated with small cell bronchial carcinoma.

Miller and Sellink (1979)[45] indicate that plain abdominal radiographs in pseudo-obstruction show distended loops indistinguishable from mechanical obstruction so that barium small bowel studies are necessary to demonstrate that there is no mechanical factor. Treatment is difficult or impossible in generalised involvement but isolated megaduodenum responds well to duodenojejunostomy (Anuras et al., 1979)[46].

## Colonic Pseudo-obstruction

Ogilvie (1948)[47] described a form of colonic dilatation without obstruction due to retroperitoneal malignancy and because of this, acute non-obstructive colonic dilatation has been called Ogilvie's syndrome. In most cases, this type of dilatation is due to reversible paralysis associated with illness in the aged (Golladay and Byrne, 1981)[48]. It has also been associated with trauma at any age (Bullock and Thomas, 1984)[49].

Nivatvongs et al. (1982)[50] suggest colonoscopy to verify the diagnosis and decompress the colon. When the patient presents with apparent intestinal obstruction, urgent contrast studies may be carried out to identify or exclude a mechanical cause (Stewart et al., 1984)[51]. Vanek and Al Salti (1986)[52] review the literature and point out that 22% of cases recur after colonic decompression. The management is largely non-operative with treatment of the underlying cause, decompression of the colon and oxygen therapy. There is a small risk of caecal rupture which requires surgery (Addison, 1983)[53].

## Other Motility Disorders

In the large bowel, many factors influence motility but sympathetic stimulation inhibits motility and parasympathetic stimulation increases motility (Ganong, 1989)[54]. The autonomic neuropathy of diabetes mellitus may cause constipation or diarrhoea (Katz and Spiro, 1966)[55]. Large bowel and anorectal involvement are serious complications of poorly controlled insulin-dependent diabetics (Ogbonnaya and Arem, 1990)[56]. Ohri et al. (1991)[57] discussed the large range of drugs which modulate the nervous balance to produce severe constipation or pseudo-obstruction. They include phenothiazines, tricyclics, anti-parkinsonian drugs, clonidine and narcotics.

Chronic intestinal motility disorders may also be produced by replacement of smooth muscle as part of a recognised disease process such as scleroderma (Poirer and Rankin, 1972)[58] or amyloidosis (Gilat and Spiro, 1968)[59].

## References


1. Christensen J (1971) The controls of gastrointestinal movements: some old and new ideas. N Engl J Med 285:85–98
2. Lluis F, Thompson JC (1988) Neuroendocrine potential of the colon and rectum. Gastroenterology 94:832–844
3. Abbasi AA, Douglass RC, Bissell GW, Chen Y (1975) Myxoedema ileus: a form of intestinal pseudo-obstruction. JAMA 234:181–183
4. Dalla Valle A (1920) Richerche istologische su di un caso du megacolon congenito. Pediatr Napoli 28:740
5. Eek S, Knutrud O (1962) Megacolon congenitum Hirschsprung. J Oslo City Hosp 12:245–270
6. Todd IP (1977) Adult Hirschsprung's disease. Br J Surg 64:311–312
7. Swenson O, Bill AAH Jr (1948) Resection of rectum and rectosigmoid with preservation of the sphincter for benign spastic lesions producing megacolon: experimental study. Surgery 24:212–220
8. Norberg KA (1964) Adrenergic innervation of the intestinal wall studied by fluorescence microscopy. Int J Neuropharmacol 3:379–382
9. Nixon HH (1984) Megacolon and other anomalies of the colon and rectum in children. In: Surgery of the anus, rectum and colon, 5th edn. J.C. Goligher (ed). Baillière-Tindall, London, pp 305–334
10. Nixon HH (1985) Hirschsprung's disease: progress in management and diagnostics. World J Surg 9:189–202
11. Fraser GC, Berry C (1967) Mortality in neonatal Hirschsprung's disease with particular reference to enterocolitis. J Pediatr Surg 2:205
12. Frank JD, Nixon HH (1979) Causes of death in Hirschsprung's disease. Analysis and conclusions for therapy. Progr Pediatr Surg 13:199–205
13. Noblett HR (1969) A rectal suction biopsy tube for use in the diagnosis of Hirschsprung's disease. J Pediatr Surg 4:406–409

14. Lake BD, Puri P, Nixon HH et al. (1978) Hirschsprung's disease. An appraisal of histochemically demonstrated acetyl cholinesterase activity in suction rectal biopsies as an aid to diagnosis. Arch Pathol Lab Med 102:244–247
15. Lawson JON, Nixon HH (1967) Anal canal pressures in the diagnosis of Hirschsprung's disease. J Pediatr Surg 2:544–552
16. Duhamel B (1960) A new operation for the treatment of Hirschsprung's disease. Arch Dis Child 35:38–39
17. Soave F (1964) A new surgical technique for the treatment of Hirschsprung's disease. Surgery 56:1007–1014
18. Canty TG (1982) Modified Duhamel procedure for treatment of Hirschsprung's disease in infancy and childhood: review of 41 consecutive cases. J Pediatr Surg 17:773–778
19. Lynn HB, Van Heerden JA (1975) Rectal myectomy in Hirschsprung's disease. Arch Surg 110:991–994
20. Doig CM (1991) Hirschsprung's disease – a review. Int J Colorectal Dis 6:52–62
21. McCredy RA, Beart RW Jr (1980) Adult Hirschsprung's disease. Results of surgical treatment at Mayo Clinic. Dis Colon Rectum 23:401–407
22. Elliott MS, Todd IP (1985) Adult Hirschsprung's disease: results of Duhamel procedure. Br J Surg 72:884–888
23. Chagas C (1916) Trypanosomîase americana: forma acuda da moléstia. Mems Inst Oswaldo Cruz 8:37
24. Ferreira-Santos R (1961) Megacolon and megarectum in Chagas' disease. Proc R Soc Med 54:1047–1053
25. Köberle F, Nador E (1956) Mal de engasgo. Z Tropenmed Parasit 7:259
26. Corrêa Netto A, Haddad J, de Azevedo PdeAV, Raia A (1962) Etiology, pathogenesis and treatment of acquired megacolon. Surg Gynecol Obstet 114:602–608
27. Haddad J (1969) Treatment of acquired megacolon by retro-rectal lowering of the colon with a perineal colostomy: modified Duhamel operation. Dis Colon Rectum 12:421–429
28. Habr-Gama A, Goffi FS, Raia A et al. (1982) Tratemento chirurgico do megacolo-operacao de Duhamel-Haddad. Revta Col Brasil Chirurg 9:25
29. Cutait DE, Cutait R (1991) Surgery of Chagasic megacolon. World J Surg 15:188–197
30. Callaghan RP, Nixon HH (1964) Megarectum: physiological considerations. Arch Dis Child 39:153–157
31. Lane RHS, Todd IP (1977) Idiopathic megacolon: a review of 42 cases. Br J Surg 64:305–310
32. Read NW, Abouzekry I, Read MT, Howell P, Ottewell D (1985) Anorectal function in elderly patients with fecal impaction. Gastroenterology 89:959–966
33. Cummings JH (1984) Constipation, dietary fibre and control of large bowel function. Postgrad Med J 60:811–819
34. Tedesco FT, Dipiro JT (1985) Laxative use in constipation. Am J Gastroenterol 80:303–308
35. Bannister JJ, Lawrence WT, Smith A, Thomas DG, Read NW (1988) Urological abnormality in young women with severe constipation. Gut 29:17–20
36. Krevsky B, Maurer AH, Fisher RS (1989) Patterns of colonic transit in chronic idiopathic constipation. Am J Gastroenterol 84:127–132
37. Kamm MA, Hawley PR, Lennard-Jones JE (1988) Outcome of colectomy for severe idiopathic constipation. Gut 29:969–973
38. Orrom WJ, Bartolo DCC, Miller R, Mortensen NJMcC, Roe AM (1991) Rectopexy is an ineffective treatment for obstructed defecation. Dis Colon Rectum 34:41–46
39. Read NW, Timms JM, Barfield LJ, Donnelly TC, Bannister JJ (1986) Impairment of defecation in young women with severe constipation. Gastroenterology 90:53–60
40. Kawimbe BM, Papachrysostomou M, Binnie NR, Clare N, Smith AN (1991) Outlet obstruction constipation (anismus) managed by biofeedback. Gut 32:1175–1179
41. Mitros FA, Schuffler MD, Teja K, Anuras S (1982) Pathologic features of familial visceral myopathy. Hum Pathol 13:825–833
42. Schuffler MD, Lowe MC, Bill AH (1977) Studies of idiopathic pseudo-obstruction. I. Hereditary hollow visceral myopathy: clinical and pathological studies. Gastroenterology 73:327–338
43. Roy AD, Bharucha H, Nevin NC, Odling-Smee GW (1980) Idiopathic intestinal pseudo-obstruction: a familial visceral neuropathy. Clin Genet 18:291–297
44. Chinn JS, Schuffler MD (1988) Paraneoplastic visceral neuropathy as a cause of severe gastrointestinal motor dysfunction. Gastroenterology 95:1279–1286

45. Miller RE, Sellink JL (1979) Enteroclysis: the small bowel enema. Radiology 4:269–283
46. Anuras S, Shirazi S, Gardner GD, Faulk DL, Christensen J (1979) Surgical treatment for familial visceral myopathy. Ann Surg 181:306–310
47. Ogilvie H (1948) Large-intestine colic due to sympathetic deprivation. A new clinical syndrome. Br Med J ii:671–673
48. Golladay ES, Byrne WJ (1981) Intestinal pseudo-obstruction. Surg Gynecol Obstet 153:257–273
49. Bullock PR, Thomas WE (1984) Acute pseudo-obstruction of the colon. Ann R Col Surg Engl 66:327–330
50. Nivatvongs S, Vermeulin FD, Fang DT (1982) Colonoscopic decompression of acute pseudo-obstruction of the colon. Ann Surg 10:15–20
51. Stewart J, Finan PJ, Courtney DF, Brennan TG (1984) Does a water-soluble contrast enema assist in the management of acute large bowel obstruction: a prospective study of 117 cases. Br J Surg 71:799–801
52. Vanek VW, Al Salti M (1986) Acute pseudo-obstruction of the colon (Ogilvie's syndrome): an analysis of 400 cases. Dis Colon Rectum 29:203–210
53. Addison NV (1983) Pseudo-obstruction of the large bowel. J R Soc Med 76:252–255
54. Ganong WF (1989) Review of medical physiology, 14th edn. Prentice-Hall International, Hemel Hempstead, pp 408–435
55. Katz LA, Spiro HM (1966) Gastrointestinal manifestations of diabetes. N Engl J Med 275:1350–1351
56. Ogbonnaya KI, Arem R (1990) Diabetic diarrhoea: pathophysiology, diagnosis and management. Arch Intern Med 150:262–267
57. Ohri SK, Patel T, Desa L, Spencer J (1991) Drug-induced colonic pseudo-obstruction. Dis Colon Rectum 34:347–350
58. Poirer TS, Rankin GB (1972) Gastrointestinal manifestations of progressive systemic scleroderma based on a review of 364 cases. Am J Gastroenterol 58:30–44
59. Gilat T, Spiro HM (1968) Amyloidosis and the gut. Am J Dig Dis 13:619–633

# 17 Volvulus

Colonic volvulus is a rotation, most commonly of the sigmoid colon and less commonly of the ileocaecal region. Bruusgaard (1947)[1] reported that colonic volvulus involved the sigmoid colon in 65% of cases, the ileocaecal region in 32% and the transverse colon in 3% of cases.

## Sigmoid Volvulus

Shepherd (1969)[2] pointed out that there was gross geographical difference in the incidence of sigmoid volvulus as a cause of large bowel obstruction: it was less than 1% in England but it was greater than 50% in Ethiopia. Shepherd reported that in England about 8% of cases had established gangrene of the colon when they presented. He further noted that there was a tendency for sigmoid volvulus to recur; approximately one third of the cases recurred after the first attack but if a second attack occurred it became even more likely that it would be followed by further episodes. Until Bruusgaard's paper, treatment of sigmid volvulus had been by operative means but he demonstrated that non-operative measures by the passage of a rectal tube at sigmoidoscopy could rectify the situation in a majority of cases and this has been the primary therapy in most Western countries since that time.

Bruusgaard found that the typical radiographic appearance of a large single dilated loop of colon was diagnostic in almost all patients. Anderson and Lee (1981)[3] reported a large series in which they noted that the majority of patients were over 65 years of age and two thirds had either a psychiatric or significant medical illness. They reported over 80% success with tube decompression. They suggest that unless the patient is medically unfit they should go on to primary sigmoid colectomy within a few days of decompression.

Bak and Boley (1986)[4] found that the recurrence rate was very high after decompression and was accompanied by a 30% mortality. For this reason they advise that in the absence of signs of gangrene, decompression should be undertaken but that resection should follow within a few days during the same hospital admission. They found this policy reduced the mortality to 6%. Peoples et al. (1990)[5] reported that a majority of these patients had psychiatric disorders and more than half were residents in long-stay care facilities. They found that few had established gangrene which required emergency resection on presentation. In approximately half of the patients only it was possible to reduce the volvulus by either the passage of a rectal tube or by flexible sigmoidoscopy. If the volvulus was not reduced, surgery was necessary and if the volvulus recurred, operation was usually undertaken. No patients under the age of 70 died but there was an overall mortality after resection of 15% and a very high mortality in those who had established gangrene. In general, they agree that resection should be carried out soon after decompression but they question this policy in the patient over the age of 70.

Udezue (1990)[6] reporting from Nigeria in the same journal, shows that the situation is entirely different in Africa. The patients were younger, none was over the age of 40, compared with the average age of 73 in Peoples' series. Ninety-five per cent of the Nigerian series had gangrene at presentation compared with 7%. For this reason intubation was not even attempted in the Nigerian series and all their patients were treated by sigmoid resection with a mortality of 17%. Udezue does not perform primary anastomosis but advises a second operation to re-establish intestinal continuity after the patient has recovered from the acute illness.

## Ileocaecal Volvulus

Wolf and Wilson (1966)[7] state that this condition occurs with an excessively mobile right colon, that the rotation is always clockwise and that it may occur as a rare complication of pregnancy. They mention that the diagnosis is difficult with ill-defined abdominal pain, vomiting and abdominal tenderness but the signs may frequently be so indefinite that surgery is delayed. Rabinovici et al. (1990)[8] review all the papers in the last 30 years and add a few cases of their own. They stress the difficulty in diagnosis and note that gangrene had occurred in about 20% of the reported cases. Barium enema was found to have a high degree of accuracy. Almost all cases reported have been treated by operation but there is no agreement about the best operative treatment. Fixation, by either caecopexy or caecotomy, resection or simple manual correction of the volvulus are all reported in significant numbers in the papers reviewed. On review, they find that the reported recurrence rate is similar for fixation procedures or simple manual reduction. For this reason, they cannot support fixation procedures, especially caecostomy which has the highest complication and mortality rate. Resection by right hemicolectomy is indicated if there is gangrene. It carries a higher mortality than either caecopexy or manual derotation but this is probably due to the fact that it has been used for high-risk cases. The advantage of resection is that recurrence cannot occur.

## Transverse Colon Volvulus

Anderson et al. (1981)[9] reviewed the literature of this extremely rare disease.

# References


1. Bruusgaard C (1947) Volvulus of the sigmoid colon and its treatment. Surgery 22:466–478
2. Shepherd JJ (1969) The epidemiology and clinical presentation of sigmoid volvulus. Br J Surg 56:353–359
3. Anderson JR, Lee D (1981) The management of acute sigmoid volvulus. Br J Surg 68:117–120
4. Bak MP, Boley SJ (1986) Sigmoid volvulus in elderly patients. Am J Surg 151:71–75.
5. Peoples JB, McCafferty JC, Scher KS (1990) Operative therapy for sigmoid volvulus: identification of risk factors affecting outcome. Dis Colon Rectum 33:643–646
6. Udezue NO (1990) Sigmoid volvulus in Kaduna, Nigeria. Dis Colon Rectum 33:647–649
7. Wolf RW, Wilson H (1966) Emergency operation for volvulus of the cecum. Review of 22 cases. Am Surg 32:96–102
8. Rabinovici R, Simanski DA, Kaplan O, Mayor E, Manny J (1990) Cecal volvulus. Dis Colon Rectum 33:765–769
9. Anderson JR, Lee D, Taylor TV, Ross AH (1981) Volvulus of the transverse colon. Br J Surg 68:179–181

# 18 Disorders of the Pelvic Floor

Included in this group of diseases are the following: idiopathic (neurogenic) incontinence, rectal prolapse, solitary rectal ulcer syndrome and idiopathic perineal pain. These conditions may be associated with disorders of the levator ani muscle and/or the internal and external sphincter ani muscles.

Parks et al. (1966)[1] suggested that many of these conditions had a common aetiology based on straining at stool with abnormal perineal descent consequent upon abnormal function in the puborectalis part of the levator ani. This alters the anorectal angle which Parks (1975)[2] considered important for the maintenance of continence. The concept has been challenged in recent years by other groups who advance evidence for the importance of sphincter function *per se* (Bartolo et al., 1986)[3]. Sensory appreciation within the rectum is equally important and Duthie and Bennett (1963)[4] brought forward the concept of a sampling zone at the anorectal junction. Disturbances in the distensibility or compliance of the rectum from inflammatory disease or surgery may also disturb continence (Buchmann et al., 1980)[5].

## Incontinence

So-called idiopathic faecal incontinence is ascribed to a traction injury to the pudendal nerve supplying the sphincter complex. This was first suggested by Parks and has been supported by studies carried out at St Mark's Hospital (Swash, 1983)[6]. The damage may be due to perineal descent but may be associated with difficult childbirth with prolonged labour in previous years (Read et al., 1984)[7]. Sphincter damage from any injury (civil, military, surgical or obstetric) may cause incontinence. A large series was reviewed in the Sir Alan Parks memorial symposium (Motson et al., 1983)[8].

The abnormalities of the pelvic floor are best investigated by a series of studies of anorectal function which include:

- Anal canal pressure measurement at rest and on straining (Duthie, 1971)[9]
- Anorectal reflex (Aaranson and Nixon, 1972)[10]
- Rectal sensation and compliance (Aaranson and Nixon, 1972)[10]
- Perineal descent (Henry et al., 1982)[11]
- Motor nerve conduction times (Kiff and Swash, 1984)[12]
- Electromyography, concentric/single fibre (Neil and Swash, 1980)[13]

- Defecating proctogram (Mahieu et al., 1984)[14]
- Intestinal transit times (for constipation)
- Endoanal ultrasound (for sphincter damage) (Law et al., 1991)[15].

A recent study involving colorectal surgeons in both the USA and the UK indicated that practising surgeons still tend to rely most on the history and clinical examination but would tend to support their observations by manometry, measurements of rectal compliance and defecography (Karulf et al., 1991)[16].

The treatment of incontinence should be conditioned by its cause. Incontinence due to sphincter damage or idiopathic incontinence are most amenable to treatment. Non-operative methods for which success has been claimed are electrical stimulation (Hopkinson and Lightwood, 1966)[17] and biofeedback (Engel et al., 1974)[18]. Surgical treatment is effective in some patients with idiopathic incontinence for which Parks (1975)[2] described the operation of postanal repair in which the anorectal angle was "restored" by coapting muscle by an operation in the intersphincteric space. Parks reported successful outcome in almost 80% of cases but others have had difficulty in achieving such a high success rate.

For incontinence due to sphincter injury, Parks and McPartlin (1971)[19] described a method of repair in which the scar tissue was excised and the divided sphincter repaired with overlap. This method has produced good results. On rare occasions a gracilis muscle sling around the anus may be indicated if a substantial part of the external sphincter is lost (Pickrell et al., 1952)[20]. Williams et al., (1991)[21] have refined this technique of gracilis transposition by using an implanted nerve stimulator to convert the muscle from a fast twitch to a slow twitch type and report encouraging success in constructing a functioning neosphincter.

## Rectal Prolapse

Sun et al. (1989)[22] suggested that rectal prolapse and solitary rectal ulcer share a common pathophysiology with a hypersensitive rectum and weak anal sphincters. Similar changes are found in both mucosal prolapse and total rectal prolapse. Although rectal prolapse occurs in children under 2 years of age it can usually be managed conservatively (Stephens, 1958)[23]. The predominant age group is the elderly in whom it should be considered as an intussusception of the rectum (Devadhar, 1965)[24]. Total rectal prolapse is commonly associated with incontinence but about 65% of patients return to acceptable continence after a successful repair (Williams et al., 1991)[25]. Although many of these patients are of advanced age they tolerate the abdominal surgery required for the correction of the prolapse well. There is little morbidity and even less mortality. Keighley et al. (1983)[26] report a series of 100 operations without an operative death. If there is recurrence it is often some years after operation (Schlinkert et al., 1985)[27].

Historically, total rectal prolapse was treated by an anal encirclement with wire or other material. The results of this were unsatisfactory and this was well demonstrated by Porter (1962)[28]. There are advocates of anterior resection (Goldberg et al., 1980)[29] but most surgeons would now use an abdominal route to fix the rectum to the sacrum. The material used is non-absorbable in these operations but since good results in controlling the prolapse have been reported by several methods, the material and the type of fixation appear to be unimportant. The successful methods include posterior fixation by polyvinyl alcohol sponge (Morgan and Wells, 1962)[30] or by Marlex mesh (Keighley et al. 1983)[26] and anterior fixation with Mersilene mesh (Ripstein, 1965)[31]. Other surgeons have used a perineal approach using Delorme's procedure, with a low recurrence rate (Uhlig and Sullivan, 1979)[32].

The chief problem after surgery is persisting incontinence but Goldberg et al. (1980)[29] observed that continence tended to improve for many months. The results of postanal repair as a secondary procedure are uncertain (Williams et al., 1991)[25].

## Solitary Rectal Ulcer Syndrome

Solitary rectal ulcer is an unusual condition and is best described as the solitary ulcer syndrome because the rectal abnormality may not show ulceration. Further, the ulceration may be multiple rather than solitary. The microscopic and clinical features are well described by Madigan and Morson (1969)[33]. The lesion is often on the anterior rectal wall and it is suggested that it may be caused by mucosal prolapse (Rutter and Riddell, 1975)[34] or incomplete intussusception (White et al., 1980)[35]. The prolapsing mucosa or intussusception is entrapped by the muscles so that it becomes engorged and ulcerates. Du Boulay et al. (1983)[36] compared the histology and mucin production in patients with solitary rectal ulcer syndrome and mucosal prolapse. They found similar histological features and a common change in the mucin from sulphomucin to sialomucin along the whole crypt. They believe that mucosal prolapse syndrome is a preferable term.

Treatment is difficult and results are inconsistent. Many patients can be managed conservatively but if a definite internal prolapse can be demonstrated then rectopexy may produce good results (Martin et al., 1981)[37]. Symptoms may justify more intrusive surgery but defunctioning colostomy and even abdominoperineal excision of the rectum leave some patients with persisting symptoms (Ford et al., 1983)[38].

## Idiopathic Anal Pain

Anal pain without demonstrable cause is difficult to categorise (Thiele, 1937)[39]. There appear to be two variants, chronic persistent pain – the levator syndrome or coccygodynia – and intermittent, more severe pain, proctalgia fugax.

It has been felt that the levator syndrome may be associated with abnormalities in the levator ani. This syndrome is ill-defined but includes anal pain radiating to the lower back or the buttocks. Sinaki et al. (1977)[40] noted that in half the patients there was radiation into the legs. At that time transanal massage of the levatores was thought to be effective treatment in many patients. The condition became referred to as the levator syndrome and Sohn et al. (1982)[41] reported that a high percentage of patients responded well to high voltage electrogalvanic stimulation. Billingham et al. (1987)[42] in a small study report that this treatment along with others helps a few patients but on follow-up after some months a majority have not benefited.

An interesting paper from France is the first systematic study of the relationship between depression and coccygodynia (Maroy, 1988)[43]. The author suggests that many of these patients have depression and in patients in whom rectal examination produced tenderness in the coccyx or adjacent muscles this is likely to be a sign of depression. He suggests that in these patients enquiry should be made for other signs of depression such as night wakening and he suggests that treatment should be with well-chosen antidepressants.

Proctalgia fugax is characterised by irregular and short-lived pelvic pain which is very severe and thought to be due to intense spasm of the rectal smooth muscle or internal sphincter or possibly the pelvic floor (Wright, 1985)[44]. Bouquet et al. (1986)[45] have suggested that the condition is produced by transient ischaemia and suggest that diltiazem, a calcium antagonist useful in vasospastic disease, is effective in relieving the condition. Swain (1987)[46] has found that clonidine, an $\alpha_2$ adrenoreceptor agonist, was useful in treatment of himself.

## References


1. Parks AG, Porter NH, Hardcastle J (1966) The syndrome of the descending perineum. Proc R Soc Med 59:477–482
2. Parks AG (1975) Anorectal incontinence. Proc R Soc Med 68:681–690
3. Bartolo DC, Roe AM, Locke-Edmunds JC, Virjee J, Mortensen NJ (1986) Flap-valve theory of anorectal incontinence. Br J Surg 73:1012–1014
4. Duthie HL, Bennett RC (1963) The relation of sensation in the anal canal to the functional anal sphincter: a possible factor in anal continence. Gut 4:179–182
5. Buchmann P, Mogg GAG, Alexander-Williams J, Allan RN, Keighley MRB (1980) Relationship of proctitis and rectal capacity in Crohn's disease. Gut 21:137–140
6. Swash M (1983) Pathophysiology of idiopathic (neurogenic) faecal incontinence. Ann R Coll Surg Engl (Suppl) 65:22–23
7. Read NW, Bartolo DCC, Read MG (1984) Difference in anal function in patients with incontinence to solids and in patients with incontinence to liquids. Br J Surg 71:39–42
8. Motson RW, McPartlin JF, Browning GGP (1983) Anal sphincter injury. Ann R Coll Surg Engl (Suppl) 65:33–35
9. Duthie HL (1971) Progress report on anal continence. Gut 12:844–852
10. Aaranson I, Nixon HH (1972) Clinical evaluation of anorectal pressure studies in the diagnosis of Hirschsprung's disease. Gut 13:138–146
11. Henry MM, Parks AG, Swash M (1982) The pelvic floor musculature in the descending perineum syndrome. Br J Surg 69:470–472
12. Kiff ES, Swash M (1984) Slowed conduction in the pudendal nerves in idiopathic (neurogenic) faecal incontinence. Br J Surg 71:614–616
13. Neil ME, Swash M (1980) Increased motor unit fibre density in the external anal sphincter

muscle in anorectal incontinence: a single fibre EMG study. J Neurol Neurosurg Psychiatry 43:343–347
14. Mahieu P, Pringot J, Bodard P (1984) Defecography. I. Description of a new procedure and results in normal patients. Gastrointest Radiol 9:247–251
15. Law PJ, Kamm MA, Bertram CI (1991) Anal endosonography in the investigation of faecal incontinence. Br J Surg 78:312–314
16. Karulf RE, Coller JA, Bartolo DCC et al. (1991) Anorectal physiology testing. A survey of availability and use. Dis Colon Rectum 34:464–468
17. Hopkinson BR, Lightwood R (1966) Electrical treatment of anal incontinence. Lancet i:297–298
18. Engel BT, Nikoomanesh P, Schuster MM (1974) Operant conditioning of rectosphincteric repairs in the treatment of faecal incontinence. N Engl J Med 290:646–649
19. Parks AG, McPartlin JF (1971) Late repair of injuries of the anal sphincter. Proc R Soc Med 64:1187–1189
20. Pickrell KL, Broadbent TR, Masters FW, Metzger JT (1952) Construction of a rectal sphincter and restoration of anal continence by transplanting the gracilis muscle. Ann Surg 135:853–862
21. Williams NS, Patel J, George BD, Hallen RI, Watkins ES (1991) Development of an electrically stimulated neoanal sphincter. Lancet 338:1166–1169
22. Sun WM, Read NW, Donnelly TC, Bannister JJ, Shorthouse AJ (1989) A common pathophysiology for full thickness rectal prolapse, anterior mucosal prolapse and solitary rectal ulcer. Br J Surg 76:290–295
23. Stephens FD (1958) Minor surgical conditions of the anus and perineum in paediatrics. Med J Aust 1:244–246
24. Devadhar DSC (1965) A new concept of mechanism and treatment of rectal procedentia. Dis Colon Rectum 8:75–77
25. Williams JG, Wong WD, Jensen L, Rothenberger DA, Goldberg SM (1991) Incontinence and rectal prolapse: a prospective manometric study. Dis Colon Rectum 34:209–216
26. Keighley MRB, Fielding JWL, Alexander-Williams J (1983) Results of Marlex mesh abdominal rectopexy for rectal prolapse in 100 consecutive patients. Br J Surg 70:229–232
27. Schlinkert RT, Beart RW Jr, Wolff BG, Pemberton JH (1985) Anterior resection for complete rectal prolapse. Dis Colon Rectum 28:409–412
28. Porter NH (1962) Collective results of operation for rectal prolapse. Proc R Soc Med 55:1087–1091
29. Goldberg SM, Gordon PH, Nivatvongs S (1980) Essentials of anorectal surgery. Lippincott, Philadelphia
30. Morgan CN, Wells C (1962) Polyvinyl alcohol sponge prosthesis. Proc R Soc Med 55:1083–1084
31. Ripstein CB (1965) Surgical care of massive rectal prolapse. Dis Colon Rectum 8:34–38
32. Uhlig BE, Sullivan ES (1979) The modified Delorme operation: its place in surgical treatment of massive rectal prolapse. Dis Colon Rectum 22:513–514
33. Madigan MR, Morson BC (1969) Solitary ulcer of the rectum. Gut 10:71–81
34. Rutter KRP, Riddell RH (1975) The solitary ulcer syndrome of the rectum. Clin Gastroenterol 4:505–530
35. White CM, Findlay JM, Price JJ (1980) The occult rectal prolapse syndrome. Br J Surg 67:528–530
36. Du Boulay CEH, Fairbrother J, Issacson PG (1983) Mucosal prolapse syndrome – a unifying concept for solitary ulcer syndrome and related disorders. J Clin Pathol 36:1264–1268
37. Martin CJ, Parks TG, Biggart JD (1981) Solitary rectal ulcer syndrome in Northern Ireland 1971–1980. Br J Surg 68:744–747
38. Ford MJ, Anderson JR, Gilmour HM, Holt S, Sircus W, Heading RC (1983) Clinical spectrum of "solitary ulcer" of the rectum. Gastroenterology 84:1533–1540
39. Thiele GH (1937) Coccygodynia and pain in the superior gluteal region and down the back of the thigh; causation by tonic spasm of the levator ani, coccygeus and piriformis muscles and relief by massage of these muscles. JAMA 109:1271–1275
40. Sinaki M, Merritt JL, Stillwell GK (1977) Tension myalgia of the pelvic floor. Mayo Clin Proc 52:717–722
41. Sohn N, Weinstein MA, Robbins RD (1982) The levator syndrome and its treatment with high-voltage electrogalvanic stimulation. Am J Surg 144:580–582

42. Billingham RP, Isler JT, Friend WG, Hostetler J (1987) Treatment of levator syndrome using high-voltage electrogalvanic stimulation. Dis Colon Rectum 30:584–587
43. Maroy B (1988) Spontaneous and evoked coccygeal pain in depression. Dis Colon Rectum 31:210–215
44. Wright JE (1985) Inhaled salbutamol for proctalgia fugax. Lancet ii:659–660
45. Bouquet J, Moore N, Lhuintre JP, Boismare F (1986) Diltiazem for proctalgia fugax. Lancet i:1493
46. Swain R (1987) Oral clonidine for proctalgia fugax. Gut 28:1039–1040

# 19 Perianal Abscess and Fistula

Perianal infection may present as an acute abscess or as a chronic discharging fistula but the two states are so interrelated that they are discussed together. These conditions have been recorded in writings for more than 2000 years. Fistulas were treated by ligatures, corrosives or laying open by the knife. John of Arderne in 1370 described the principles of surgical treatment which accord with modern ideas (Power, 1910)[1].

Acute abscess formation around the anal canal may be related to infection from the skin or from the anal canal. Studies of the bacteriology of pus from these infections have been shown to be useful in defining the site of origin (Grace et al., 1982)[2]. Most abscesses and fistulas are of anal origin and although some may complicate a fissure, most are due to infection in an anal gland (Eisenhammer, 1958)[3]. Parks (1961)[4] demonstrated multiple anal glands each draining into an anal crypt. The opening into the crypt is at the same site as the internal opening of a fistula. This work supported the theory that perianal infection was commonly due to infection in an anal gland. The glands lie between the internal and external sphincters and infection originates in this area in most perinanal abscesses and fistulas. Similarly, this concept is the basis of classification and treatment. The abscess starts in the intermuscular plane but usually spreads to the perianal region as a perianal abscess. If it spreads to present in the ischiorectal area the patient is more toxic and may be dangerously ill (Abcarian, 1976)[5]. Less common abscesses are submucous or pelvirectal.

Treatment of the acute abscess may be carried out as a one- or two-stage procedure. The one-stage operation consists of draining the abscess and at the same time finding the internal opening and laying the tract open. A large series reporting good results by this technique is reported by McElwain et al. (1966)[6] The two-stage procedure involves drainage of the abscess and follow-up to determine the possible subsequent development of a fistula. Classically drainage was followed by packing the cavity as a routine, the results of which are well documented (Buchanan and Grace, 1973)[7]. Recently it has become realised that complex aftercare is unhelpful. Goldberg et al. (1980)[8] drain the abscesses under local anesthesia as an outpatient procedure. Others suggest drainage and insertion of a small "mushroom" drain (Isbister, 1989)[9]. The rate of fistula formation after simple drainage varies from less than 20% to more than 60% (Goligher, 1984)[10].

Fistula-in-ano commonly follows an anorectal abscess. The condition requires an understanding of the anal anatomy and pathophysiology for treatment. For this reason, complex classifications have been proposed from time to time. Goodsall (1900)[11] laid down his rule which states that if a transverse line is drawn across the middle of the anus any fistula opening anterior to that line will run straight to the nearest crypt, whilst if the opening is posterior to the line the tract will be curved and enter the posterior midline crypt. This rule is true for many fistulas but there are many exceptions. More important is the disposition in relationship to the anal musculature. Earlier classifications were flawed due to anatomical misconceptions. A better understanding of the anatomy led to the modern classification proposed by Parks et al. (1976)[12]. The majority of the fistulas are below puborectalis and are classified as either low intersphincteric, traversing the internal sphincter only or transsphincteric traversing the lower part of both sphincters. The higher fistulas which have a definite relationship to the puborectalis are rare but are subdivided into high transsphincteric, suprasphincteric and extrasphincteric. In the absence of previous surgery or bowel disease fistulas do not communicate with the rectum (Goligher, 1984)[10].

Marks and Ritchie (1977)[13] report a large series of fistulas and show that there is a male preponderance. They classify the fistula by the Parks method and report on the results of treatment. The majority of patients had low fistulas which were cured by operation with a low incidence of minor disturbances of continence. The complex and high fistula had less satisfactory results. Many had some disturbance in continence and a few were incontinent even to a solid stool. The usual method of treatment is to lay open a low fistula and allow the wound to heal by granulation which produces excellent results (Shouler et al., 1986)[14]. Tracts traversing the sphincter muscles high in the anal canal are much more difficult to manage. Parks and Stitz (1976)[15] used a loose seton as a "drain" in high fistula and left it in situ for 3 months or more. It was removed after drainage ceased and they report excellent results. Williams et al. (1991)[16] summarise various methods for high fistula and report their experience with tight "cutting" setons and a loose seton plus two-stage fistulotomy. Mann and Clifton (1985)[17] proposed a different method of dealing with the high fistula in that they dissected out the tract and transposed it entirely into the intersphincteric space after dividing and then repairing the external sphincter. The newly positioned fistula is then laid open or excised at a second operation. Jones et al. (1987)[18] reported on the use of transanal rectal advancement flaps to treat fistula-in-ano and rectovaginal fistula. For high fistula-in-ano the internal opening and surrounding tissue is excised and a broad-based rectal flap is brought down to cover the defect. The external tracts are laid open or excised sparing the rectal musculature. Many of these patients had Crohn's disease but the procedure was satisfactory in 60% of the patients with Crohn's rectovaginal fistula as compared with 80% of the non-Crohn's rectovaginal fistulas. It was successful in complex anorectal fistulas in one third of the patients with Crohn's disease and in all the patients who did not have Crohn's disease. Wedell et al. (1987)[19] report the use of a similar technique with a rectal advancement flap and coring out the external tract in the treatment of a high fistula. They report that the operation produced healing in all of the 27 patients treated. The last two papers stress that the rectal flap should be thick and contain some muscular tissue. Other methods such as primary grafting (Hughes, 1953)[20] and exploration of the intersphincteric space with excision of the affected gland with coring out of external tracts (Parks, 1961)[4] have not been widely accepted. Seow-Choen and Nicholls (1992)[21] give a comprehensive review of anal fistula. The care of these patients after operation has changed in recent years from regular packing by the nursing staff to a policy of self-caring with minimal supervision which allows sound and rapid healing (Hughes et al., 1983)[22].

The very rare rectal fistulas require temporary colostomy and closure of the rectal defect to produce satisfactory results (Marks and Ritchie, 1977)[13].

## Unusual Causes of Perianal Sepsis

### Crohn's Disease

Penna and Crohn (1938)[23] recognised that perianal fistula and anal canal ulceration were commonly associated with Crohn's disease. Morson and Lockhart-Mummery (1959)[24] noted that anal Crohn's disease may precede bowel disease and in some instances remained localised for many years. It is still believed by many that the surgical treatment of anal canal Crohn's disease should be ultra-conservative (Allan and Keighley, 1988)[25] but Marks et al. (1981)[26] showed that successful fistula surgery could be carried out in patients with quiescent Crohn's disease and Hobbiss and Schofield (1982)[27] showed that the healing rate after surgery for a low fistula was similar in patients with or without Crohn's disease.

### Hidradenitis Suppurativa

Woollard (1930)[28] defined the apocrine gland areas in the axillae, groins and perianal region. Hidradenitis suppurativa is characterised by infective sinuses in these glandular areas. Jackman and McQuarrie (1949)[29] indicated that the perineum was involved alone in about one third of cases. Wiltz et al. (1990)[30] in a recent publication presented a retrospective review and advocate treatment by wide local excision. They point out that it is a difficult condition to treat but have not found skin grafting useful. This is in contrast to many other groups (Goligher, 1984)[10]. It is a condition which produces diagnostic difficulty. In particular, it can be confused with perianal Crohn's disease (Goligher, 1984)[10]. It is a disease which tends to recur and Morgan and Hughes (1979)[31] suggested that a sweat test by appropriate stimulation of the apocrine area would allow exact mapping by starch and iodine powder. It is hoped that by accurate demarcation the results of radical surgery will be improved.

### Pilonidal Sinus

Allen-Mersh (1990)[32] reviews in great detail pilonidal sinus lying in its usual sacrococcygeal position posterior to the anus. The article discusses incidence, pathogenesis, pathology and clinical features and exhaustively reviews the results of various types of treatment.

Rarely pilonidal sinus can occur in other clefts such as the umbilicus and the axilla. Of particular interest have been the reports of pilonidal sinus in the interdigital clefts of barbers (Patey and Scarff, 1948)[33].

## Tuberculosis

Tuberculous infection can present as a fistula-in-ano without other evidence of the disease. This manifestation is rare in Western communities but is seen more commonly in areas where tuberculosis is endemic (Gilinsky et al., 1983)[34]. Anal infection and ulceration are also seen in relationship to sexually transmitted diseases. This has been increasingly reported with the increase in HIV infection by Safavi et al. (1991)[35] who reviewed this subject.

# References


1. Power D (1910) Treatise of fistula-in-ano, haemorrhoids and clysters by John Arderne. Oxford University Press, Oxford
2. Grace RH, Harper IA, Thompson RG (1982) Anorectal sepsis: microbiology in relationship to fistula-in-ano. Br J Surg 69:401–403
3. Eisenhammer ST (1958) A new approach to the anorectal fistulous abscess based on the high intermuscular lesion. Surg Gynecol Obstet 106:595–599
4. Parks AG (1961) Pathogenesis and treatment of fistula-in-ano. Br Med J i:463–469
5. Abcarian H (1976) Acute suppuration of the anorectum. In: Surgical annual 8. L.H. Nyhus (ed). Appleton-Century-Crofts, New York, p 103
6. McElwain JW, Alexander RM, MacLean MD (1966) Primary fistulectomy for anorectal abscess: clinical study of 500 cases. Dis Colon Rectum 9:181–185
7. Buchanan R, Grace RH (1973) Anorectal suppuration: the results of treatment and the factors influencing the recurrence rate. Br J Surg 60:537–540
8. Goldberg SM, Gordon PH, Nivatvongs S (1980) Essentials of anorectal surgery. Lippincott, Philadelphia
9. Isbister WH (1989) A simple method for the management of anorectal abscess. Aust NZ J Surg 57:721–724
10. Goligher JC (1984) Surgery of the anus, rectum and colon, 5th edn. Baillière Tindall, London, p 174
11. Goodsall DH (1900) Diseases of the anus and rectum. Longman, London
12. Parks AG, Gordon PH, Hardcastle JD (1976) A classification of fistula-in-ano. Br J Surg 63:1–12
13. Marks CG, Ritchie JK (1977) Anal fistulas at St. Mark's Hospital. Br J Surg 64:84–91
14. Shouler PJ, Grimley RP, Keighley MRB, Alexander-Williams J (1986) Fistula-in-ano is usually simple to manage surgically. Int J Colorect Dis 1:113–115
15. Parks AG, Stitz RW (1976) The treatment of high fistula-in-ano. Dis Colon Rectum 19:489–499
16. Williams JG, MacLeod CA, Rothenberger DA, Goldberg SM (1991) Seton treatment of high anal fistula. Br J Surg 78:1159–1161
17. Mann CV, Clifton MA (1985) Re-routing of the track for the treatment of high anal and anorectal fistula. Br J Surg 72:134–137
18. Jones IT, Fazio VW, Jagelman DG (1987) The use of transanal rectal advancement flaps in the management of fistulas involving the anorectum. Dis Colon Rectum 30:919–923
19. Wedell J, Meier zu Eissen P, Banzhaf G, Kleine L (1987) Sliding flap advancement for the treatment of high level fistulae. Br J Surg 74:390–391
20. Hughes ESR (1953) Primary skin-grafting in proctological surgery. Br J Surg 41:639–642
21. Seow-Choen F, Nicholls RJ (1992) Anal fistula. Br J Surg 79:197–205

22. Hughes ESR, Cuthbertson AM, Killingback MK (1983) Anorectal suppuration II: anal fistula. pp 142–162 In: Colorectal surgery. Churchill Livingstone, Edinburgh
23. Penna A, Crohn BB (1938) Perianal fistulas as a complication of regional ileitis. Ann Surg 108:867–873
24. Morson BC, Lockhart-Mummery HE (1959) Anal lesions in Crohn's disease. Lancet ii:1122–1125
25. Allan A, Keighley MRB (1988) Management of perianal Crohn's disease. World J Surg 12:198–202
26. Marks CG, Ritchie JK, Lockhart-Mummery HE (1981) Anal fistulas in Crohn's disease. Br J Surg 68:525–527
27. Hobbiss JH, Schofield PF (1982) Management of perianal Crohn's disease. J R Soc Med 75:414–417
28. Woollard HH (1930) Cutaneous glands of man. J Anat 64:415–421
29. Jackman RJ, McQuarrie HB (1949) Hidradenitis suppurativa: its confusion with pilonidal disease and anal fistula. Am J Surg 77:349–351
30. Wiltz O, Schoetz DJ, Murray JJ, Roberts PL, Coller JA, Veidenheimer MC (1990) Perianal hidradenitis suppurativa. Dis Colon Rectum 33:731–734
31. Morgan WP, Hughes LE (1979) The distribution, size and density of the apocrine glands in hidradenitis suppurativa. Br J Surg 66:853–856
32. Allen-Mersh TG (1990) Pilonidal sinus: finding the right track for treatment. Br J Surg 77:123–132
33. Patey DH, Scarff RW (1948) Pilonidal sinus in a barber's hand with observations on postanal pilonidal sinus. Lancet ii:13–14
34. Gilinsky NH, Marks IN, Kottler RE, Price SK (1983) Abdominal tuberculosis in a ten-year review. South Afr Med J 64:849–857
35. Safavi A, Gottesman L, Dailey TH (1991) Anorectal surgery in the HIV+ patient: update. Dis Colon Rectum 34:299–304

# 20 Anal Fissure

Acute and chronic anal fissure are well described in the literature of the nineteenth century. As long ago as 1865, Lane[1] described the hypertrophied polyp at the upper end of a fissure. The aetiology of a simple anal fissure is uncertain; it has been ascribed to injury in passing hard faeces (Ball, 1908)[2] or cryptitis (Buie and Butsch, 1938)[3]. The chronic fissure is most usually in the posterior midline associated with sphincter spasm and pain. Klosterhalfen et al. (1989)[4] have suggested a reason for this posterior predisposition as being ascribed to a lessened blood supply from the inferior rectal artery to the posterior part of the anal canal. This type of supply occurs in 85% of patients, which tallies well with the frequency of the distribution of fissure in this quadrant of the anal canal.

Treatment of the condition in the acute phase may be by conservative methods using local anaesthetic creams. Traditionally it was suggested that a small dilator should be passed daily but this has been shown to produce no improvement in results (McDonald et al., 1983)[5]. The chronic fissure is treated by operative means under local or general anaesthesia. Dilatation of the anal canal was first described by Racamier[6] in 1838 but is still practised with moderate success in the treatment of fissure. Earlier this century, injection of longlasting local anaesthetic had a vogue but has now fallen out of use (Yeomans et al., 1927)[7].

The principal procedure currently in use is the operation of internal sphincterotomy. Surprisingly the first reference to this was in 1818 by Boyer[8]. Gabriel (1948)[9] advised excision of the fissure with division of the tissue deep to this. Eisenhammer (1951)[10] showed that this divided tissue was the lower part of the internal sphincter. From this knowledge, a less radical operation of division of the lower sphincter fibres in the base of the posterior fissure was introduced (Eisenhammer, 1953)[11]. Bennett and Goligher (1962)[12] reviewing the results of this procedure, showed that about 30% of patients had minor defects in continence due to a posterior fibrous track, the "keyhole deformity" (Duthie and Bennett, 1964)[13]. Eisenhammer (1959)[14] suggested that lateral internal sphincterotomy would avoid this and produce less functional disturbance. This was confirmed by Hoffman and Goligher (1970)[15], who showed that only 7% of patients had very minor disturbance of continence after this procedure. Lateral sphincterotomy may be performed as an open operation but similar results are produced with the lesser approach of subcutaneous lateral internal sphincterotomy, as described by Notaras (1969)[16].

Lewis et al. (1988)[17] have compared open and closed internal sphincterotomy. They found no significant difference in the rate of healing or morbidity with either method and no differences between local and general anaesthesia. Six per cent of fissures either failed to heal or recurred in a series of 350 patients who had been followed for at least 14 months. Eight patients (2.3%) had developed wound infection or low level fistula. There was minor incontinence in 17% but in a majority this was transient. Minor incontinence lasting for longer than 6 weeks occurred in only 6%.

## References


1. Lane JR (1865) Clinical observations on disease of the rectum. II. On polypoid growths in the rectum and their occasional association with anal fissure. Lancet ii:87–88
2. Ball C (1908) The rectum: its diseases and developmental defects. Frowde, Hodder and Stoughton, London
3. Buie LA, Butsch WL (1938) The importance of recognising contracted anus. Am J Dig Dis Nutr 5:162–164
4. Klosterhalfen B, Vogel P, Rixen H, Mittermayer C (1989) Topography of the inferior rectal artery: a possible cause of chronic primary anal fissure. Dis Colon Rectum 32:43–52
5. McDonald P, Driscoll AM, Nicholls RJ (1983) The anal dilator in the conservative management of acute anal fissures. Br J Surg 70:25–26
6. Racamier JC (1838) Extension, massage et percussion cadencée dans le traitment des contractures musculaires. Rev Méd Fr Estrang 1:74–89
7. Yeomans FC, Gorsch RV, Mathesheimer JL (1927) Benacol in the treatment of pruritus ani. Trans Am Proctol Soc 28:24–29
8. Boyer A (1818) Remarques et observations sur quelques maladies de l'anus. J Compl Dict Sci Méd 2:24
9. Gabriel WB (1948) Principles and practice of rectal surgery, 4th edn, H.K. Lewis, London, pp 173–177
10. Eisenhammer ST (1951) The surgical correction of chronic internal anal contracture. South Afr Med J 25:486–489
11. Eisenhammer ST (1953) The internal anal sphincter: its surgical importance. South Afr Med J 27:266–270
12. Bennett RC, Goligher JC (1962) Results of internal sphincterotomy for anal fissure. Br Med J ii:1500–1503
13. Duthie HL, Bennett RD (1964) Anal sphincteric pressure in fissure in ano. Surg Gynecol Obstet 119:19–21
14. Eisenhammer ST (1959) The evaluation of the internal anal sphincterotomy operation with special reference to an anal fissure. Surg Gynecol Obstet 109:583–590
15. Hoffman DC, Goligher JC (1970) Lateral subcutaneous internal sphincterotomy in treatment of anal fissure. Br Med J iii:673–675
16. Notaras MJ (1969) Lateral subcutaneous sphincterotomy for anal fissure: a new technique. Proc R Soc Med 62:713
17. Lewis TH, Corman ML, Prager ED, Robertson WG (1988) Long-term results of open and closed sphincterotomy for anal fissure. Dis Colon Rectum 31:368–371

# 21 Haemorrhoids

For centuries, haemorrhoids were considered to be analogous to varicose veins of the anal canal but this hypothesis is now known to be inaccurate. Thomson (1975)[1] by careful anatomical dissection and clinical observation has shown that internal haemorrhoids are related to normal vascular cushions in the anal canal. These cushions are distensible and can be controlled by local fibromuscular tissue (Thomson, 1979)[2]. Haemorrhoids are a displacement or hypertrophy of these cushions. The displacement can lead to bleeding, prolapse or thrombosis. It is ill understood why these normal structures become disturbed but Hancock (1977)[3] has produced some evidence that patients may have an abnormality in the internal sphincter though more recently there has been suggestion that the observed pressure increases are due to the increased bulk of the cushions in the anal canal. Burkitt (1979)[4] has suggested that the prevalence of internal haemorrhoids is due to a low residue diet and has advocated a high-fibre diet as a method of management. External haemorrhoids are swellings distal to the dentate line. These are painful and described by many as perianal haematomata but the thrombosis may be within a perianal venous space (Thomson, 1982)[5]. If seen early after their onset they may be excised. They resolve possibly leaving tags, which may cause irritation and require removal.

Schofield (1981)[6] amongst others, pointed out that when a patient presents complaining of haemorrhoids a full history and examination is required to exclude more serious disease such as carcinoma of the rectum or inflammatory bowel disease. It was stressed that treatment of haemorrhoids should be appropriate to the symptoms and that many patients would respond to simple conservative management. Surgical management of piles by ligation, excision or cautery has been used since ancient times (Schofield,1981)[6]. In the nineteenth century injection of sclerosants into the piles was introduced and achieved popularity (Anderson, 1924)[7]. For many years, injection treatment with 5% phenol in almond oil introduced into the submucosa above the pile, was the treatment of choice for minor internal piles (Morley, 1928)[8]. Haemorrhoidectomy was advised for all other degrees of internal piles. In the last 25 years a number of minor methods of treatment of internal piles have been advocated. These can be carried out as outpatient procedures and include anal dilatation as proposed by Peter Lord (1969)[9], elastic band ligation, popularised by Barron (1963)[10] and further refined by Hulton and Schofield (1984)[11] or cryosurgery using freezing by nitrous oxide (Williams et al., 1973)[12] or liquid nitrogen (Lewis, 1972)[13]. At least two further minor methods of treatment have been added in recent years with satisfactory short-term results. Neiger (1979)[14] has suggested infrared coagulation and

Griffith et al. (1987)[15] have suggested bipolar diathermy coagulation. None of these methods seems to produce as good a long-term result as formal haemorrhoidectomy but may be justified because they are successful in the majority of patients in the medium term and produce less disturbance for the patient. Various trials have been conducted of the different methods of treatment and a number of these are reviewed by Nicholls and Glass (1985)[16]. The older established method of injection of sclerosants now has a relatively limited place but formal haemorrhoidectomy still produces the best results and is justified for severe problems with haemorrhoids.

Grace and Creed (1975)[17] have shown that haemorrhoidectomy is the preferred method for prolapsed, strangulated haemorrhoids. Formal haemorrhoidectomy may be carried out by the open method with the low ligation of Milligan and Morgan (1937)[18] or a high ligation or a closed method as pioneered by Ferguson and Heaton (1959)[19]. The open method, carried out under general anaesthesia in the lithotomy position is favoured in the UK whereas the closed method, carried out in the jackknife position under local or regional anaesthesia, is favoured in many centres in the United States. Roe et al. (1987)[20] compared open and closed haemorrhoidectomy and showed no clinical difference in the results. Wang et al. (1991)[21] report the results of using Nd-YAG laser for internal haemorrhoids and $CO_2$ laser for external haemorrhoids and report satisfactory results on short-term follow-up with a shorter hospital stay and a lesser complication rate when compared with closed haemorrhoidectomy. The present practice in the treatment of internal and external haemorrhoids is well summarised in a paper by the Standards Task Force of the American Society of Colon and Rectal Surgeons (1990)[22].

## References


1. Thomson WHF (1975) The nature of haemorrhoids. Br J Surg 62:542–552
2. Thomson WHF (1979) The anal cushions – a fresh concept in diagnosis. Postgrad Med J 55:403–405
3. Hancock BD (1977) The internal sphincter and the nature of haemorrhoids. Gut 18:651–655
4. Burkitt DP (1979) Epidemiological features. In: Haemorrhoids, current concepts on causation and management. International congress and symposium 12. C. Wood (ed). Royal Society of Medicine, London, pp 3–9
5. Thomson WHF (1982) The real nature of "perianal haematoma" Lancet ii:467–468
6. Schofield PF (1981) Comparative studies of different methods of treatment. In: The haemorrhoid syndrome. H.D. Kaufman (ed). Abacus Press, Tunbridge Wells, pp 145–153
7. Anderson HG (1924) The injection method for the treatment of haemorrhoids. Practitioner 113:399–409
8. Morley AS (1928) An improved technique for the treatment of internal haemorrhoids by injection. Lancet i:543–545
9. Lord PH (1969) A day case procedure for the cure of third degree haemorrhoids. Br J Surg 56:747–749
10. Barron J (1963) Office ligation of internal haemorrhoids. Am J Surg 105:563–570
11. Hulton N, Schofield PF (1984) Elastic band ligation of haemorrhoids: a new applicator. Br J Surg 71:212
12. Williams KL, Haq IV, Elem B (1973) Cryodestruction of haemorrhoids. Br Med J i:666–668

13. Lewis IM (1972) Cryosurgical hemorrhoidectomy. A follow-up report. Dis Colon Rectum 15:128–134
14. Neiger A (1979) Haemorrhoids in everyday practice. Proktologie 1:22
15. Griffith CDM, Morris DL, Ellis I et al. (1987) Outpatient treatment of haemorrhoids by bipolar diathermy coagulation. Br J Surg 74:827
16. Nicholls RJ, Glass R (1985) In: Coloproctology. Springer, Berlin, Heidelberg, New York, p 92
17. Grace RH, Creed A (1975) Prolapsing thrombosed haemorrhoids: outcome of conservative management. Br Med J iii:354
18. Milligan ETC, Morgan C, Naughton Jones LE, Officer R (1937) Surgical anatomy of the anal canal and the operative treatment of haemorrhoids. Lancet ii:1119–1124
19. Ferguson JA, Heaton JR (1959) Closed haemorrhoidectomy. Dis Colon Rectum 2:176–179
20. Roe AM, Bartolo DCC, Vellacott KD, Locke-Edmunds, Mortensen NJMcC (1987) Submucosal versus ligation excision haemorrhoidectomy. A comparison of anal sensation, anal sphincter manometry and postoperative pain and function. Br J Surg 74:948–953
21. Wang JY, Chang-Chien CR, Chen J-S, Lai C-R, Tang R (1991) The role of lasers in hemorrhoidectomy. Dis Colon Rectum 34:78–82
22. American Society of Colon and Rectal Surgeons, Standards Task Force (1990) Practice parameters for the treatment of hemorrhoids. Guideline article. Dis Colon Rectum 33:992–993

# 22 Pruritis Ani

Perianal itching may be due to an anal or rectal abnormality, vaginal discharge, dermatological disease or it may be idiopathic. Alexander (1975)[1] discusses the dermatological causes which include fungal infection and candidiasis with or without vaginal discharge. Bowyer and McColl (1966)[2] identify erythrasma due to infection with *Candida minutissimum* as an unusual cause. Alexander-Williams (1983)[3] highlights the danger of allergy to local anaesthetic creams used in the treatment of pruritis which may produce acute worsening of the condition.

Threadworm (pinworm) infestation often presents as pruritis ani which tends to be nocturnal but is easily treated with piperazine (Brown et al., 1956)[4]. The idiopathic variety of pruritis ani has been attributed to the leakage of alkaline material onto the perianal skin (Heslop, 1966)[5]. Support for an increased tendency to leakage came from Eyers and Thomson (1979)[6] who found that patients with pruritis had abnormal anal manometry. Allan et al. (1987)[7] confirmed the presence of abnormal anal physiology in these patients; in particular, they found an abnormal fall in anal pressure in response to rectal dilatation with a balloon.

When dermatological, gynaecological or local anal cause is found then treatment is directed to this. Murrie et al. (1981)[8] showed that if pruritis coexisted with haemorrhoids the pruritis was improved or eliminated by treatment of the haemorrhoids. Treatment of the idiopathic variety is difficult. Alexander-Williams (1985)[9] has laid down the principals of management with emphasis on some simple measures of hygiene. Some cases may be intractable and various operative methods have been advocated for these patients. In general, the results have been disappointing but recently the perianal injection of methylene blue is said to have produced good results (Eusebio et al., 1990)[10].

## References


1. Alexander S (1975) Dermatological aspects of anorectal disease. Clin Gastroenterol 4:651–657
2. Bowyer A, McColl I (1966) The role of erythrasma in pruritus ani. Lancet ii:572–573
3. Alexander-Williams J (1983) Pruritus ani. Br Med J 287:159–160
4. Brown HW, Chan KF, Hussey KL (1956) The treatment of enterobiasis and ascariasis with piperazine. JAMA 161:515–520
5. Heslop JH (1966) Primary pruritus ani. Dis Colon Rectum 9:119–120

6. Eyers AA, Thomson JPS (1979) Pruritus ani: is anal sphincter dysfunction important in aetiology? Br Med J ii:1549–1551
7. Allan A, Ambrose NS, Silverman S, Keighley MRB (1987) Physiological study of pruritus ani. Br J Surg 74:576–579
8. Murrie JA, Sim AGW, MacKenzie I (1981) The importance of pain, pruritus ani and soiling as symptoms of haemorrhoids and their response to haemorrhoidectomy or rubber band ligation. Br J Surg 68:247–249
9. Alexander-Williams J (1985) Pruritus ani – what to do, what not to do, to control this infernal itch? Postgrad Med J 77:56–65
10. Eusebio EB, Graham J, Mody N (1990) Treatment of intractable pruritus ani. Dis Colon Rectum 33:770–772

# 23 Anal Tumours

## Benign Tumours

The commonest benign tumour of the perianal region and the anal canal is viral in origin and takes the form of multiple warts or condyloma acuminata. These have been recognised from ancient times (Oriel, 1971)[1]. They are often associated with vulval or penile warts (Abcarian et al., 1976)[2]. They are shown to contain intranuclear inclusion bodies (Oriel and Almeida, 1970)[3] and have been shown to be associated with papilloma virus (Frazer et al., 1986)[4].

Many series show a high incidence of anoreceptive homosexuality (Oriel, 1971)[1] and may be associated with rectal venereal disease. Malignant transformation can occur but is rare (Lee et al., 1981)[5].

Treatment is difficult because of a tendency to reinfection but immunisation with a vaccine prepared from excised wart tissue has been shown to be effective in a high percentage of cases (Abcarian et al., 1976)[2].

Local treatment by a cytotoxic chemical, podophyllin, may be used. Physical destruction by diathermy, cryosurgery or cautery has been practised for years but produces pain and stenosis if the lesions are widespread (Goligher, 1984)[6]. The preferred method of local treatment appears to be scissor excision (Thomson and Grace, 1978)[7]. This causes few local symptoms but there may be recurrence from reinfection.

## Malignant Tumours

Morson and Sobin (1976)[8] put forward the classification of tumours agreed by the World Health Organization (WHO). The tumours are classified into those below the dentate line, called anal margin tumours and those above the dentate line, called anal canal tumours. Although the anal canal can be involved from downgrowth of a rectal adenocarcinoma the commonest malignant tumour is a squamous cell carcinoma with its variants, the basaloid or cloacogenic and the mucoepidermoid carcinoma. The commonest anal margin tumour is also the squamous cell carcinoma but rare tumours include the basal cell carcinoma, Bowen's disease, Paget's disease and malignant melanoma. Thus, squamous cell carcinomas are separated into tumours of the anal canal and tumours of the anal verge. The latter have a slightly better prognosis after appropriate wide excision (Stearns and Quan, 1970)[9]. Anoreceptive homosexual behaviour seems to be a predisposing factor in some patients especially if they are immunosuppressed by HIV (Lorenz et al., 1991)[10]. Recent studies have shown the association of papilloma virus with a majority of these tumours (Palmer et al., 1988)[11]. In females with anal carcinoma, carcinoma of the cervix is more likely to develop and is also associated with papilloma virus. Fenger (1991)[12] describes a modification to WHO classification where the anal canal above the dentate line is subdivided into the anal transitional zone and the colorectal region. He discusses the predisposing factors and the histopathology of the varieties of anal tumour.

Treatment was for many years either wide local excision for the anal verge tumour or abdominoperineal excision of the anal canal and rectum for the anal canal tumours. Some centres used interstitial radiotherapy or external beam radiotherapy (Papillon, 1988)[13]. In recent years the picture has changed with the introduction of chemotherapy and radiotherapy combined regimes with apparently much improved results. The development of this method is reviewed by the innovator, Dr Nigro (Nigro, 1991)[14]. In the UK, this combined therapy is, at present, the subject of a comparative trial against radiotherapy alone (Northover, 1991)[15]. The tumour tends to metastasise late and distant metastases are relatively rare (Gordon, 1990)[16]. Lymph node metastases occur in the inguinal nodes and markedly worsen the prognosis especially if the involved nodes are apparent at presentation (Stearns and Quan, 1970)[9]. Involved nodes can be treated by either radiotherapy or block dissection of the groin, and the latter appears to produce the better results (Stearns and Quan, 1970)[9].

## Rare Anal Tumours

The subject of anal neoplasms is well reviewed by Gordon (1990)[16]. Of particular interest is Bowen's disease, which has a typical appearance and is an intraepithelial squamous carcinoma. Beck et al. (1988)[17] review the situation and recommend excision and grafting or a rotation flap repair. Berardi et al. (1988)[18] describe perianal Paget's disease which is an intraepithelial adenocarcinoma arising from apocrine glands. This has a tendency to local malignancy and coexistent visceral malignancy (Jensen et al., 1988)[19]. Malignant melanoma is another rare tumour, which is well reviewed by Goldman et al. (1990)[20]. It responds very poorly even to the most radical of treatments (Ward et al., 1986)[21].

# References


1. Oriel JD (1971) Anal warts and anal coitus. Br J Venereal Dis 47:373–376
2. Abcarian H, Smith D, Sharon N (1976) The immunotherapy of anal condyloma acuminatum. Dis Colon Rectum 19:237–244
3. Oriel JD, Almeida JE (1970) Demonstration of virus particles in human genital warts. Br J Venereal Dis 46:37–42
4. Frazer IH, Medley G, Crapper RM, Brown TC, Mackay IR (1986) Association between anorectal dysplasia, human papillomavirus and human immunodeficiency virus in homosexual men. Lancet ii:657–660

5. Lee SH, McGregor OH, Kuziez MN (1981) Malignant transformation of perianal condyloma acuminatum: a case report with review of the literature. Dis Colon Rectum 24:462–467
6. Goligher JC (1984) Surgery of the anus, rectum and colon, 5th edn. Baillière Tindall, London
7. Thomson JPS, Grace RH (1978) Treatment of perianal and anal condylomata acuminata: a new operative technique. J R Soc Med 71:180–185
8. Morson BC, Sobin LH (1976) Histologic typing of intestinal tumours. World Health Organization, Geneva, pp 62–65
9. Stearns MW, Quan SH (1970) Epidermoid carcinoma of the anorectum. Surg Gynecol Obstet 151:953–957
10. Lorenz HP, Wilson W, Crombleholme T, Schecter W (1991) Squamous cell carcinoma of the anus and HIV infection. Dis Colon Rectum 34:336–338
11. Palmer JC, Shepard NA, Jass JR et al. (1988) Human papillomavirus type 16 in anal squamous carcinomas. Lancet ii:42
12. Fenger C (1991) Anal neoplasia and its precursors: facts and controversies. Semin Diagn Pathol 8:190–201
13. Papillon J (1988) Current therapeutic concepts in management of carcinoma of the anal canal. Cancer Res 110:146–149
14. Nigro ND (1991) The force of change in the management of squamous cell cancer of the anal canal. Dis Colon Rectum 34:482–486
15. Northover J (1991) Epidermoid cancer of the anus – the surgeon retreats. J R Soc Med 84:389–390
16. Gordon PH (1990) Current status: perianal and anal canal neoplasms. Dis Colon Rectum 33:799–808
17. Beck DE, Fazio VW, Jagelman DG, Lavery IC (1988) Perianal Bowen's disease. Dis Colon Rectum 31:419–422
18. Berardi RS, Lee S, Chen HP (1988) Perianal extramammary Paget's disease. Surg Gynecol Obstet 167:359–366
19. Jensen SL, Sjolin KE, Shokough-Amiri MH, Hagen K, Harling H (1988) Paget's disease of the anal margin. Br J Surg 75:1089–1092
20. Goldman S, Glimelius B, Pahlman L (1990) Anorectal malignant melanoma in Sweden: report of 49 patients. Dis Colon Rectum 33:874–877
21. Ward MW, Roman G, Nicholls RJ (1986) The surgical treatment of anorectal malignant melanoma. Br J Surg 73:68–69

# Subject Index

# Author Index